NUTRITIONAL SUPPORT IN
HOSPITAL PRACTICE

Nutritional Support in Hospital Practice

D. B. A. SILK
MD, FRCP
Consultant Physician,
Central Middlesex Hospital,
London

FOREWORD BY

SIR FRANCIS AVERY JONES
CBE, MD, FRCP, Hon. FRCS (Lond.),
MD (Melb.), Hon D. Univ (Surrey)
Consulting Physician,
Central Middlesex Hospital, London,
Honorary Consulting Physician,
St Bartholomew's Hospital, London,
Consulting Gastroenterologist,
St Mark's Hospital, London,
Emeritus Consultant in Gastroenterology
to the Royal Navy

BLACKWELL SCIENTIFIC PUBLICATIONS

OXFORD LONDON
EDINBURGH BOSTON MELBOURNE

© 1983 by
Blackwell Scientific Publications
Editorial offices:
Osney Mead, Oxford, OX2 OEL
8 John Street, London WC1N 2ES
9 Forrest Road, Edinburgh EH1 2QH
52 Beacon Street, Boston,
  Massachusetts 02108, USA
99 Barry Street, Carlton
  Victoria 3053, Australia

First published 1983

Set and printed at The Alden Press, Oxford
Bound by Cambridge University Press

DISTRIBUTORS

USA
  Blackwell Mosby Book Distributors
  11830 Westline Industrial Drive
  St Louis, Missouri 63141

Canada
  Blackwell Mosby Book Distributors
  120 Melford Drive, Scarborough
  Ontario M1B 2X4

Australia
  Blackwell Scientific Book Distributors
  214 Berkeley Street, Carlton
  Victoria 3053

British Library Cataloguing in Publication
Data

Silk, D. B. A.
  Nutritional support in hospital practice.
  1. Nutrition   2. Diet in diseases
  I. Title
  612'.3   RM216

ISBN 0-632-01105-X

Contents

	Foreword	vi
	Preface	vii
1	Introduction	1
2	The Nutritional Team	5
3	Diagnosis of Malnutrition	9
4	Indications for Nutritional Support	27
5	Metabolic Responses to Starvation and Injury	42
6	Nutritional Requirements and Methods of Providing Nutritional Support	51
7	Enteral Feeding	68
8	Parenteral Feeding	102
9	The Liver and Nutrition	150
10	The Kidney and Nutrition	166
	Index	179

Foreword

This timely book shows the contribution which clinical nutrition can make to improving patient care in hospitals. Until antibiotics were developed the combination of poor nutrition and infection contributed to the significantly high mortality and morbidity associated with many hospital admissions, particularly for patients needing surgical operations. Nowadays, infections can be largely overcome and this has highlighted the dangers of poor nutrition to patients with poor nutrition, and also the adverse role it plays in many patients with serious illnesses. Today, so much more can be done both in the assessment and control of sub-optimal nutrition in hospitals. The introduction of chemically defined foods for astronauts led on to the development of parenteral feeding, which has such life-saving potential for many seriously ill patients. More recently it has become appreciated, in large measure due to the studies undertaken by Dr David Silk, that new techniques of enteral feeding can provide an invaluable measure of support for those who have become very debilitated, particularly necessary when they need an operation.

Translating knowledge into practice is always a difficult administrative, as well as clinical, exercise. It is here that the nutrition assessment team can make an outstanding contribution. Such teams bring together clinical, nursing, pathology and the pharmacy services, and are of special significance not only in ensuring appropriate and prompt treatment but also in achieving a high cost-effectiveness. The greater interest in nutrition within hospital practice is rapidly being reflected in the recognition of the need to take more action in educating the public and particularly those who can influence others, such as teachers.

The practical application of clinical nutrition is easily and appropriately grafted on the gastroenterology department, with its special experience of the problems of absorption and malabsorption in the gut. Nevertheless, other hospital departments, such as cardiology, surgery, paediatrics, metabolic and geriatrics, can provide a leadership. It seems likely that within the next decade every hospital will have organised an effective clinical nutrition service.

Preface

There was no formal clinical nutritional service when I arrived at the Central Middlesex Hospital. This is not to say that the patients were being denied nutritional support. Patients receiving enteral nutrition were however being fed a variety of diets by a variety of techniques and patients receiving parenteral nutrition were receiving a variety of different regimes depending largely on the ward that they were in. It also appeared to me that some patients who needed nutritional support were not being treated and vice versa and that few attempts were being made to monitor the efficacy of treatment. Moreover little note was being made of nitrogen and energy requirements of the individual patient and the complication rates, particularly in parenterally fed patients, seemed to be unduly high.

During the last four years we have attempted to rationalise clinical nutrition throughout the hospital. A close rapport has been achieved between the Pharmacy, Dietetic Department, the nursing staff, the Departments of Chemical Pathology and Bacteriology and above all else with my Medical and Surgical colleagues throughout the hospital. A closely knit nutritional team has evolved from this collaboration and as a result I think the nutritional care of our patients has improved.

This book is thus largely based on the experiences gained by the nutrition team at the Central Middlesex Hospital and I am very pleased to have the opportunity to thank many of my colleagues who have helped us so much. Dr Peter Frost, Consultant Chemical Pathologist has provided us with invaluable assistance in the nutritional care of all patients we have treated. Without the efforts of the late Mr Horney, Chief Pharmacist at Central Middlesex Hospital, it would have been impossible to rationalise parenteral nutrition in the way that we have, and I am most grateful to all past and present members of the Dietetic Department and Nursing Staff who have given us so much support throughout. I am particularly grateful for the support, enthusiasm and close cooperation I have received from my consultant colleagues, in particular Drs Martin McNicol, John Riordan, George Misiewicz, Stewart McHardy-Young, Mr John Newcombe, Mr Robin Illingworth, Mr Martin Rice-Edwards, Mr Neil Menzies-Gow and Mr Michael Henry. I would like to pay a special personal tribute to my two research fellows Drs Barry Jones and Patrick Keohane who between them have been primarily responsible for looking after all aspects of the nutritional care of patients we have treated.

I would like to thank Sir Francis Avery-Jones for the support he has given me throughout and for his contribution to this book. I would also like to thank Mrs Mary Lang who has helped me so much with the bibliography, Mrs Dawn Sayers, Mrs Linda Rimmer and Miss Denise Western have most efficiently provided secretarial help, Mr Adam Sisman has provided me with friendly and very patient and highly professional guidance throughout.

Finally I would like to dedicate this book to my wife Heather and children Jennie, Rachael, Emma and James, without whose encouragement and support the project would have never been completed.

Chapter 1
Introduction

It has been known for over 40 years that patients who have lost more than 20% of their body-weight carry a higher risk of developing post-operative complications and have a higher mortality than those who have lost less weight [1]. Although the dangers of weight loss, particularly in surgical patients, remained an acknowledged fact, nearly 30 years passed before the first prospective clinical surveys were published suggesting that malnutrition in hospital medicine is a much wider problem than had previously been considered.

Thus, 30–50% of patients in medical and surgical wards in hospitals in the USA and the UK are now known to have evidence of nutritional deficiencies [2–6]. That the nutritional needs of the hospitalised patient had been a much neglected aspect of clinical management for many years is not now in dispute, nor is there any doubt that one of the main reasons for this has been the lack of emphasis placed on nutrition in the medical curriculum [7]. In my view, other reasons why so few advances were made in clinical nutrition in hospital medicine include the widespread resistance amongst physicians and surgeons for using the methods then available, and the lack of enthusiasm for developing new techniques for providing nutritional support.

Despite the fact that it has been common knowledge for years that the basic energy requirements of man are in the region of 1500–2000 calories per day, standard practice has been to provide 1–2 litres of 5% dextrose to hospitalised patients who are unable to eat. Simple calculations will reveal that such a regime will provide a maximum of 400 calories a day.

Basic concepts of clinical nutrition in hospital medicine can be developed from this statement. Thus, in simplistic terms, the deficit between energy requirements and intake has to be made up from energy drawn from body reserves. As carbohydrate energy reserves are minimal, body protein and fat has to be broken down to provide energy, with the result that weight is lost and the patient wastes away.

We know from recent experiences of the hunger strikers in the Maze prison in Belfast that if intake of nutrients is completely withheld man can survive for 40–60 days [8]. In the majority of hospitalised patients, however, energy requirements are in excess of those of simple starvation, and death will ensue far earlier. Moreover, there are even greater dangers that can occur to the sick hospitalised patient who is faced with prolonged starvation; profound hypoproteinaemia interferes with wound healing [9] and increases the susceptibility of the patient to shock [10] as well as increasing susceptibility to excess salt and water intake [11]. Furthermore, alterations in body constituents, particularly in respect of protein stores, have been shown to correlate with increased susceptibility to infection [12], all of which will hasten the demise of these patients.

In the light of these comments, it is hoped that the reader will be convinced that malnutrition in the hospitalised patient does have major clinical consequences, some of which are summarised in Table 1.1.

Table 1.1   Clinical consequences of protein calorie malnutrition [14].

Loss of body weight
Diminished muscle mass
Hypoproteinaemic oedema
Impaired immunocompetence—humoral and cellular
Increased susceptibility of infection
Poor wound healing; dehiscence
Apathy
Increased mortality

Definitions of malnutrition

Often clinicians are confused about the definitions used to describe malnutrition and some of the terms require clarification.

The term *protein calorie malnutrition* or *protein energy malnutrition* (PEM) was introduced to dispel the earlier exclusive emphasis on protein lack in the aetiology of malnutrition of the kwashiorkor type and give appropriate emphasis to calorie deficiency in nutritional disorders. PEM thus embraces all disorders attributable to a lack of protein and calories, including marasmus and kwashiorkor, and frequently serves as a euphemism for starvation.

Although those interested in malnutrition in the world's population, particularly in underdeveloped countries, continue to search for an accepted classification of PEM in order to provide a basis for comparing differences in prevalance and pathogenesis of marasmus and kwashiorkor [13], such a step would not appear to be necessary in hospital medicine. As one is dealing with patients who have reduced intakes of protein and energy, the terms protein calorie or protein energy malnutrition will quite adequately describe the type of malnutrition that occurs in adult hospitalised patients seen in most hospitals in the developed countries.

The realisation that malnutrition is common in hospital medicine has come at a time of rapid developments in techniques of providing nutritional support. It is therefore within the power of the average clinician to prevent the progression of malnutrition in their patients. The clinical importance of malnutrition will continue to increase in the future because of the emergence of multiple devices to support failing organ systems. Moreover, the use of such devices has allowed prolonged hospitalisation, often with multiple episodes of stress.

The overall aim of this book is, therefore, to increase the practising clinician's knowledge of nutrition and to create an awareness that malnutrition is a definable medical syndrome that by and large will respond to appropriate therapy.

REFERENCES

1 Studley H.O. (1936) Percentage of weight loss; basic indicator of surgical risk in patients with chronic peptic ulcer. *J. Am. Med. Assoc.* **106**, 458.
2 Bistian B.R., Blackburn G.L., Hallowell E. & Heddle R. (1974) Protein status of general surgical patients. *J. Am. Med. Assoc.* **235**, 1567.
3 Bistian B.R., Blackburn G.L., Vitale J., Cochrane D. & Naylor J. (1976) Prevalance of malnutrition in general medical patients. *J. Am. Med. Assoc.* **235**, 1567.
4 Hill G.L., Pickford I., Young G.A., Schorah C.J., Blackett R.L., Burkinshaw L., Warren J.V. & Morgan D.B. (1977) Malnutrition in surgical patients: An unrecognised problem. *Lancet* **i**, 689.
5 Leevy C.M., Cardi L., Frank O., Gellene R. & Baker H. (1965) Incidence and significance of hypovitaminaemia in a randomly selected municipal hospital population. *Am. J. Clin. Nutr.* **17**, 259.
6 Bollet A.J. & Owens S. (1973) Evaluation of nutritional status of selected hospitalised patients. *Am. J. Clin. Nutr.* **26**, 931.
7 Butterworth C.E. (1974) The skeleton in the hospital closet. *Nutrition Today* **9**, 4.
8 Love A.H.G. (1982) Prolonged starvation. In *Extremes of Nutrition.* First British Society of Gastroenterology/Glaxo International Teaching Day.
9 Rhoads J.E. (1975) In *Manual of Surgical Nutrition*, eds. W.F. Ballinger, J.A. Collins, W.R. Drucker *et al*, p. 4. W.B. Saunders, Philadelphia.

10 Rardin I.S., MacNamee H.G., Kamholz J.H. & Rhoads J.E. (1944) Effect of hypoproteinaemia on susceptibility to shock resulting from haemorrhage. *Arch. Surg.* **48**, 491.

11 Wilmore D.N. (1977) *The metabolic management of the critically ill*, p. 174. Plenum Medical, New York.

12 Koehane P.P., Attrill H., Jones B.J.M., Brown I., Frost P. & Silk D.B.A. (1983) The roles of lactose and *C. difficile* in the pathogenesis of enteral feeding associated diarrhoea. *Clin. Nutr.* (in press).

13 James W.P.T. (1982) Assessement of Nutritional Status. *Med. Int.* **1**, 660.

14 Lee H.A. (1979) Why Enteral Nutrition? *Res. Clin. Forums* **1**, 15.

Chapter 2
The Nutritional Team

As this book will show, nutritional support now involves the use of specialised equipment and techniques that are tending to become increasingly complex and expensive. Moreover some of the procedures, such as catheter insertion for parenteral feeding, carry a significant morbidity and mortality.

Since the outset of our nutritional programme we have recognised that to obtain maximum efficiency and safety in the use of these specialised techniques, close cooperation between all the disciplines involved in clinical nutrition is essential. To formalise this relationship throughout our hospital the concept of the nutritional support team was evolved. In our particular case the team has included those interested and closely involved in clinical nutrition, and we would recommend that the composition and policy aims of nutritional support teams established elsewhere should be tailored to facilities and requirements within that particular hospital.

Overall aims

Table 2.1 summarises the overall aims of a nutritional support team. Before the composition of a nutritional support team is decided upon it is important to clarify the ground rules for the service. A decision has to be made as to whether a single group is going to provide advice about nutritional support throughout the whole hospital, or whether different groups of individuals will provide advice for different departments, for example a team headed by an anaesthetist providing nutritional support in the intensive care unit and a surgically-orientated team providing nutritional support for all surgical patients, etc. Our own experience has been based upon the establishment of the nutrition team that advises all members of staff throughout the hospital, and it is our belief that this is the most satisfactory method as it facilitates rationalisation of equipment and standardisation of clinical techniques throughout the whole hospital. As a result of this we have not only been able to reduce expenditure on equipment but we have also been able to achieve

Table 2.1   Suggested aims of the nutrition team.

Define local politics of the nutritional service

Rationalise equipment

Standardise clinical technique

Education

Research

Table 2.2   Suggested composition of nutrition team.

Consultant clinician

Consultant clinical pathologist

Senior pharmacist

Senior dietitian

Specialised nutrition nurse

Physiotherapist

a financial saving in the purchase of enteral diets and nutrient solutions for parenteral nutrition by bulk ordering. The establishment of a nutrition team that is responsible for advising about nutritional care throughout the hospital obviously necessitates close cooperation between all consultant colleagues, an aim that we were easily able to achieve at Central Middlesex Hospital.

We believe that the nutrition support team should play a major role in the education of clinical and nursing colleagues and we lay great emphasis on this: I think there is general agreement that patient care has benefitted from such an approach.

In our unit we have from the outset had a keen interest in clinical research. The establishment of a rationalised nutrition programme should make simple clinical research possible in any District General hospital.

Personnel

The suggested composition of the nutritional support team is shown in Table 2.2. In our experience a consultant clinician, consultant clinical pathologist, senior pharmacist, and a senior dietitian will all play an important role. We would suggest that these members be permanent staff in order to provide continuity of service and teaching for Junior staff.

While the involvement of an experienced clinician is essential to provide experitise and advice, this central role can be performed by any consultant who has an interest in clinical nutrition, e.g. a general physician, gastroenterologist, surgeon or anaesthetist.

As the clinical pathology department will be responsible for estimations of nitrogen balance, nutritional parameters and biochemical monitoring, particularly in those patients receiving parenteral nutrition, a close cooperation with the consultant clinical pathologist is important. Catheter-related sepsis remains a problem with parenteral nutrition, so a close liaison with the bacteriology department has proved to be a necessity.

The senior pharmacist will be responsible for storage and preparation of nutrient solutions for parenteral nutrition together with preparation of 3-litre bags, if facilities are available; his close cooperation is therefore clearly essential. The senior dietitian and her staff will provide expertise relating to enteral 'sip' or tube feeding as well as specialised enteral diets. Depending on the type of diet prescribed the dietetic department may also be responsible for diet and container preparation. The senior dietitian thus becomes an important member of the nutritional support team.

In addition, close involvement of other personnel may be very useful. The physiotherapist for example can provide considerable assistance when mobilising malnourished patients and, as outlined in Chapter 8, cooperation of a surgeon skilled at insertion of central feeding lines for parenteral nutrition is essential.

Even more topical is the employment of a specially trained nutrition nurse who would have responsibility for nursing care in respect of the technical side of enteral and parenteral nutrition. There is now evidence (see Chapter 8) that care of parenteral feeding catheters by a specially trained nutrition nurse results in a significant reduction in the incidence of catheter sepsis and in our experience the employment of such a nurse provides greater scope for teaching of nursing staff about the general management of patients receiving nutritional support, as well as teaching nurses about such procedures as nasogastric tube insertion at ward level.

Role of the nutrition team within the hospital

The major role of the nutrition team is to be available for advice or to coordinate management of patients thought to require nutritional support. This simplifies the management problems facing medical and nursing staff involved with any malnourished patient. Additionally, rationalisation of equipment used on the wards will not only simplify nutritional therapy, but often reduces cost while at the same time increasing safety. It should be re-emphasised that the extent of involvement both within individual units and with individual patients must depend on cooperation with attending clinicians and this in turn often depends on providing the services that they require.

Chapter 3
Diagnosis of Malnutrition

As mentioned in Chapter 1 a number of recent studies have suggested that up to 20–50% of hospitalised patients with medical and surgical disorders have some clinical, biochemical, haematological or immunological evidence of protein calorie malnutrition [1–5]. This suggests in turn that awareness of the nutritional status of patients is a neglected area of clinical management, a situation that has been traced back to the lack of emphasis placed on clinical nutrition in the medical curriculum [6].

Two important questions arise from the above statement. Firstly, how do we diagnose protein calorie malnutrition in hospitalised patients and, secondly, even if there is agreement that the patient is malnourished does this have sufficient clinical consequences to warrant institution of nutritional support, with its attendant complications, as well as the financial burdens that it places on health care.

RECOGNITION AND DIAGNOSIS OF PROTEIN CALORIE MALNUTRITION

Nutritional assessment is the first essential step in the adequate nutritional care of any patient. Few problems arise in recognising the grossly malnourished patient (Fig. 3.1): weight loss is marked and muscle-wasting extreme. Serum albumin levels may be as low as 20 g/l and hypoproteinaemic oedema may be present. Problems arise, however, in reaching the diagnosis in the fitter-looking patients who at first sight may even look obese (Fig. 3.2). In these patients simple bedside impressions of nutritional status are invariably erroneous [7].

During the last few years a battery of clinical, biochemical, haematological and immunological tests have been described as aids to reaching a diagnosis of protein calorie malnutrition. However, by and large, when faced with these tests, the average clinician becomes uncertain about which is the most appropriate and confused as to their role in the overall management of the patient [8]. The author certainly shares this viewpoint, so the aim of this chapter is to produce a balanced view of the value of these tests in the diagnosis of protein calorie malnutrition. Table 3.1 summarises the subgroups of different investigations that are available.

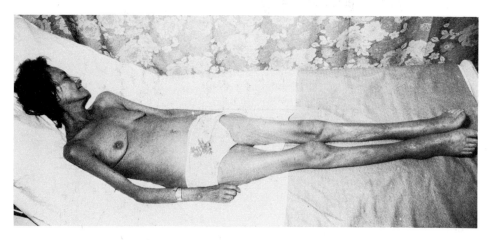

Fig. 3.1. Obvious protein calorie malnutrition in a 44-year old lady admitted for investigation of diarrhoea and abdominal pain and found to have extensive Crohn's disease. Note the marked muscle wasting and hyperproteinaemic oedema of the ankles. Serum albumin 25 g/l.

Clinical and dietary history

In clinical practice, the critical factor initiating nutritional assessment is awareness of the possibility that the patient may be wasted [9]. A routine clinical history usually neglects nutritional intake and a specific dietary history may be most valuable in directing the clinician immediately toward the possible diagnosis of protein calorie malnutrition [10]. In our unit, for example, we have been quite surprised to find that patients randomised to controlled clinical trials of enteral nutrition have had a markedly reduced nutrient intake for at least 2 weeks before nutritional support was instituted [11, 12]. Finally, when performing estimates of nutrient intake, the possibility of nutrient malabsorption should always be considered [13, 14].

Clinical examination

Many nutritional deficiencies are unaccompanied by physical signs, but clinical examination should always be carried out. Angular stomatitis, increased capillary fragility, anaemia, muscle wasting and oedema signify severe nutritional deficiency.

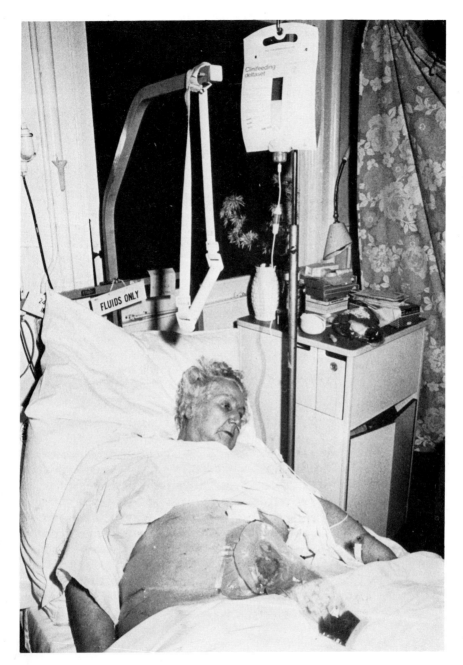

Fig. 3.2. Severe protein calorie malnutrition, but less obvious clinically (Mrs S.B. aged 65 years). Wound dehiscence and enterocutaneous fistula following second laparotomy for recurrent small bowel obstruction. Note apparent obesity. Serum albumin 24 g/l. Patient is receiving nutritional support via the enteral route.

Table 3.1 Diagnosis of protein calorie malnutrition.

Parameter	Values suggestive of protein calorie malnutrition
Clinical and dietary history	
Clinical examination	
Body weight	loss >10% normal weight
Anthropometric measurements	
Mid-arm circumference	<23 cm ♂, 22 cm ♀
Mid-arm muscle circumference	<19 cm ♂, 17 cm ♀
Skinfold thickness	see Table 3.2
Measurements of protein stores	
24-hour urinary creatinine ⎫ Creatinine height index ⎬	See Table 3.3
3-methyl histidine excretion	
Circulating hepatic proteins	
Albumin	<35 g/l
Transferrin	<2 g/l
Prealbumin	<200 mg/l
Retinol-binding protein	<100 mg/l
Immunological testing	
Lymphocyte count	<1200/mm^3
Delayed hypersensitivity skin testing	see Table 3.4

Body-weight

A significant proportion of patients admitted to general surgical and medical wards are not routinely weighed on admission. This is shortsighted because loss of body-weight may provide the first clue that a patient is malnourished and we attach importance to a loss of more than 10% of normal body-weight. Although some authors discuss the relevance of loss of 'optimal' weight (e.g. ideal weight-for-height obtained from life insurance tables), we have found this of limited value. Similarly, the body mass index (W/H^2, where W is the weight in kilograms and H the height in metres), has been shown to correlate with body fat [13]. It should also be remembered that body-weight values are meaningless in patients who are either dehydrated or, for various reasons, have fluid retention.

ANTHROPOMETRIC MEASUREMENTS

Anthropometric measurements, such as arm muscle circumference and triceps skinfold thickness (TSF) and derivates of these, have been extensively used in world surveys as a public health index of protein calorie malnutrition in children and these measurements have gained increasing importance in establishing the protein and fat reserves of hospitalised patients [1, 15, 16]. In clinical practice it has been suggested that the absolute size of muscle mass can be assessed by means of the midarm muscle circumference (MMC). This is calculated from the midarm circumference and triceps skinfold thickness, from the formula:

$$MMC = midarm\ circumference - (\pi \times triceps\ skinfold\ thickness)$$

Erroneous measurements can be obtained in oedematous patients and, contrary to expectations, correlations between changes in body nitrogen and midarm circumference and midarm muscle circumference have been shown to be poor [17], an observation with which we are in agreement.

It is now known that body fat can be estimated very simply and quickly using Harpenden skin callipers to measure skinfold thickness at four sites (Table 3.2). The sum of the four skinfolds should be greater than 40 mm. In our experience, skinfold measurements are again meaningless in obese patients and those with peripheral oedema, and we have failed to demonstrate any significant change in this parameter during either enteral [11] or parenteral feeding (B.J.M. Jones & D.B.A. Silk, pers. obs.).

Table 3.2 Measuring skinfold thickness [13].

Sites	
Triceps	Over back of left arm, at a level halfway between the acromial and olecranon processes
Biceps	At same level as triceps but anterior, with arm resting relaxed and supine
Subscapular	Over wing of left scapula, in plane of dermatome
Supra-iliac	10 mm above the left superior iliac crest in midaxillary line and along the horizontal plane

Technique
Pull all subcutaneous tissue away gently but firmly from muscle with middle finger and thumb of left hand. Maintain pressure and apply callipers with right hand 10 mm away from left hand. Maintain pressure on skinfold with left hand, release pressure on handle of callipers. Read once needle stopped moving or within 3 seconds. Repeat three times and take the two closest readings.

Equipment
Harpenden callipers obtainable from Holtain Ltd, Crosswell, Crymych, Dyfed, Wales, UK.

MEASUREMENTS OF PROTEIN STORES

Malnutrition is associated with a reduction in total body protein content and, in clinical practice, measurements of muscle mass have been regarded as relatively sensitive measures of total body protein. Midarm muscle circumference, as described above, is the simplest measure available.

The 24-hour output of urine creatinine gives a biochemical measure of muscle mass. The creatinine is derived predominantly from spontaneous cycling of creatinine phosphate in muscle at a rate of 2% of the creatinine phosphate pool per day [13]. Ingested cooked meat leads to a spurious increase in creatinine output, because the creatine phosphate content of the meat is converted into creatinine. The reference values are shown in Table 3.3, and 1 g creatinine output is taken to be derived from 20 kg muscle. Values of 70% less than normal are probably indicative of pronounced muscle wasting and below 60% severe wasting.

The creatinine–height index (CHI) is calculated by expressing the 24 hour creatinine output as a percentage of the mean value, which varies with height. Values below 80% are abnormal and values below 50% indicate severe muscle wasting.

Other more direct measures of lean body mass are available and include neutron activation analysis for whole body nitrogen, whole body counts of potassium, and isotope techniques for measuring total exchangeable potassium and body water content. These are, however, primarily of research rather than practical clinical interest.

Similarly tissue synthesis rates may be accurately measured by estimating whole body protein turnover by constant rate of infusion of ^{14}C-leucine, ^{13}C-leucine or ^{15}N-glycine. Again, we consider these to be primarily research techniques.

Table 3.3 Reference values of urinary creatinine excretion in relationship to height. Calculated from [59].

Height	Creatinine (mmol/l)	
	Males	Females
150	99	75
155	106	81
160	113	86
165	120	91
170	127	97
175	135	102
180	142	108
185	150	115
190	158	121

Finally, a great deal of interest has surrounded the measurement of 3-methylhistidine as a means of assessing the degree of muscle breakdown. When released 3-methylhistidine is not reutilised in protein synthesis and is excreted unchanged in the urine. On occasions we have felt the need to use this parameter in difficult cases, but analysis is not easy. The excretion of 4.2 μmol of 3-methylhistidine represents the breakdown of 1 g of mixed muscle protein [18].

INDIRECT MEASUREMENTS OF PROTEIN SYNTHESIS RATES

Numerous claims have been made that measurement of circulating hepatic proteins provides useful information about nutritional status, and response to nutritional support. In the absence of parenchymal liver disease and proteinuria, the serum albumin concentration provides useful information about the nutritional state, values below 30 g/l indicating moderate-to-severe malnutrition. Although claims have been made of its value in monitoring the response to treatment [19], albumin has a long half-life and, in our experience [11], as well as that of others, shows a poor response to short-term nutritional support [20]. The stability of serum albumin concentrations, despite treatment, is partly explained by the large total albumin mass, but also by the fact that hepatic synthesis of albumin may be maintained even when protein intake is restricted, as well as catabolism being reduced [21].

Transferrin has a half life of 8 days [22], shorter than albumin, and plasma levels are reduced in obvious protein calorie malnutrition [23]. We have shown that plasma levels rise in response to treatment, although this is not a universal finding [23]. Its usefulness in clinical practice is limited by co-existing iron deficiency states which promote its synthesis, and in patients who are infected and undergoing stress as part of the 'acute phase' protein response [24].

Thyroxin-binding prealbumin (TBPA) and retinol-binding protein (RBP) are two hepatic proteins whose plasma levels are also reduced in obvious protein calorie malnutrition [23]. TBPA has a half life of 2 days [25] and RBP of 12 hours [26], and theoretically both would be expected to respond to changes in nitrogen and energy input as occur during the nutritional therapy of malnourished patients. Studies indicate, though, that TBPA levels are more sensitive to changes in energy rather than nitrogen intake [20]. Plasma levels of RBP on the other hand alter rapidly in response to changes in both energy and nitrogen intake

[20], so if close monitoring of nutritional support is required in the clinical setting, plasma RBP, when measured regularly, should provide valuable information.

IMMUNOLOGICAL TESTING

Protein calorie malnutrition has now been frequently shown to be associated with impaired immunocompetence [27–29]. Based on this, immunological tests are frequently being performed as a means of monitoring treatment, and as a pre-operative test to predict post-operative morbidity and mortality.

A reduction in the total peripheral lymphocyte count to below $1200/mm^3$ is seen in obvious protein calorie malnutrition [30]. In our experience, lymphocyte counts tend to rise during nutritional therapy, although no significant changes were noted after a period of enteral nutrition, when the patient groups were considered as a whole [11]. We have, however, noted significant elevations in lymphocyte counts after parenteral nutrition (B.J.M. Jones and D.B.A. Silk, pers. obs.). Circulating T lymphocyte counts are difficult to measure, but do respond more readily to refeeding [13].

Negative skin testing with ubiquitous antigens has been frequently reported in patients with protein calorie malnutrition and skin testing has been proposed as a practical aid to the diagnosis of protein calorie malnutrition.

Skin testing should be performed by trained personnel, and the patient re-examined after 2 days. Each antigen is injected intradermally at 25 mm intervals or more, on the ventral aspect of the forearm (see Table 3.4).

We have confirmed that patients with obvious protein calorie malnutrition have negative skin tests (i.e. are anergic), as well as

Table 3.4 Cutaneous delayed hypersensitivity skin testing in adults.

Antigen	Intradermal dose
Candida	0.1 ml 1 in 100 dilution
Trichophyton	0.1 ml 1 in 100 dilution
Tuberculin	0.1 ml 1 in 100 dilution
Streptokinase–streptodornase	5 IU
Mumps	2 colony forming units

The diameter of the induration is measured 48–72 hours later; a positive reaction is recorded if the induration exceeds 5 mm in diameter patients with less obvious clinical malnutrition. We have not, however, been able to confirm the observations of others [31] that effective nutritional support is associated with reversal of the anergic state. In this respect it is important for the reader to be aware of other data showing that ageing, cancer, sarcoidosis, infection, shock and trauma have all been shown to be associated with anergy *per se*, irrespective of nutritional status [27–29, 32–35]. To this list can also be added zinc deficiency [36] and H2 receptor antagonist therapy (B.J.M. Jones, and D.B.A. Silk, pers. obs.) as well as iron [37] and folate deficiency [13].

Other immunological tests not yet in routine clinical use include measurements of immunoglobulin levels, the concentration of secretory IgA in salivary fluid, the concentration of serum C3 and microbicidal capacity testing of neutrophils, all of which show a decrease in malnutrition.

VITAMIN DEFICIENCIES

Many standard texts of clinical nutrition lay great emphasis on vitamin deficiencies. In our judgement, the relevance of vitamin deficiencies in the clinical setting, especially in respect of diagnosing protein calorie malnutrition, has been over-emphasised. Clinical features of vitamin deficiencies are unusual and, when present, reflect very severe deficiency. Nevertheless, the signs should be sought during examination. Lesser degrees may be identified by biochemical assays (Table 3.5), many of which are not in routine clinical use at present. They may become more available in the future.

DEVELOPMENT OF 'NUTRITIONAL INDICES'

Notwithstanding the drawbacks of many of the so-called nutritional indices described above, several groups have developed multiple regression computer programs to derive composite indices of nutritional status [38–40]. Combinations of serum albumin, transferrin and the anthropometric indices appear to be the most powerful aids to the diagnosis of malnutrition. It could be argued, though, that protein calorie malnutrition, the final product of the equation, remains a subjective phenomenon, so any attempt to quantify it has to be open to major criticism, particularly in cases of 'subclinical malnutrition' depicted in Fig. 3.2.

Table 3.5 Assessment of vitamin status. Data from [13].

Nutrient	Method	Normal levels	Subnormal	Deficient	Comment
Vitamin A	Serum retinol	20 μg/dl	10–19	<10	Visual dark adaptation test used for mild cases. Large vitamin A reserves in liver. Plasma level affected by binding protein concentrations which are reduced in malnutrition
Thiamine	Thiamine pyrophosphate stimulation of erythrocyte transketolase activity	1.00–1.23		>1.23	Units are relative activity with and without thiamine pyrophosphate. Needs assaying within few days
Riboflavin	Erythrocyte glutathione reductase activity stimulated by flavine adenine dinucleotide	1.0–1.2	1.2–1.4	>1.4	Enzyme activity more stable in frozen state. Clinical signs likely if >1.80
Pyridoxine	Erythrocyte glutamic-oxaloacetate transaminase stimulated by pyridoxal phosphate	1.15–1.19	—	>1.89	
Niacin	Urine N-methyl nicotinamide				Not very reliable
Folate	Serum folate	6.0 μg/ml	3.0–5.9	<3.0	Markedly affected by recent diet
	Red cell folate	160 μg/ml	140–159	<140	
Vitamin B12	Marrow deoxyuridine suppression test				
	Serum vitamin concentration	>160 ng/litre	100–159	<100	Concentrations can increase in liver disease and general malnutrition because of redistribution of hepatic stores and increase in serum transport protein concentrations
Vitamin C	Leucocyte ascorbic acid	15 μg/10^8 cells	9–15	<8	Needs 12–15 ml blood and rapid processing
Vitamin D	25-hydroxycalciferol (25-OHD)	7.5–50 mg/ml			Wide seasonal range of normal: 25-OH D affected by sunlight, diet and reserves, 1.25(OH)$_2$D assay newly introduced
	1.25-dihydroxycalciferol (1.25-(OH)$_2$D) concentrations	21–45 pg/ml	<20	<10	
Vitamin E	Serum tocopherol concentration	0.5–1.5 mg/dl			Depends on lipids. Deficient if <1.0 mg total tocopherol per gram lipids
Vitamin K	Prothrombin time	11–16 seconds	—	>17	Affected by liver disease and drugs

Ideally, measurement of the nutritional parameters discussed above should not only provide information about the diagnosis of protein calorie malnutrition, but serial measurements should also provide information about the effectiveness of nutritional support. Finally, it would be of immense value if clinically useful measures of malnutrition could be established that reliably predict post-operative complications. It is our feeling that an unreasonable burden of expectation has been placed on the use of these nutritional parameters.

Aids to diagnosis of protein calorie malnutrition

Although the methods for detecting protein calorie malnutrition have been emphasised above, many of the parameters in common use have their disadvantages.

Full clinical and dietary history-taking may, for example, not be possible in the unconscious or very ill patient. Measurement of body weight may be of limited use in oedematous or dehydrated patients. Similarly, erroneous measurements of midarm circumference, midarm muscle circumference or skinfold thickness can be obtained in oedematous patients, and the latter can also give misleading results in oedematous and obese patients.

Although hypoalbuminaemia has been claimed to accurately reflect malnutrition [41], its use can be limited by maintenance of hepatic albumin synthesis when protein intake is restricted, as well as by a reduction in its catabolism [21]. The uses of the alternative serum protein markers also have their drawbacks; transferrin, for example, is unreliable in co-existing iron deficiency anaemia and in patients who are infected and undergoing stress as part of the 'acute phase' protein response [24].

The two shorter half-life hepatic proteins, thyroxin-binding prealbumin and retinol-binding protein may be too sensitive to reductions in intake of energy and calories to be of use in diagnosing 'border line' but established cases of protein calorie malnutrition.

Finally, in respect of skin testing, it has been our experience that not all patients with obvious long-standing protein calorie malnutrition have negative responses and, as mentioned above, an 'anergic' state, as evidenced by negative skin testing, has been observed in a number of different clinical conditions irrespective of nutritional state [13, 27–29, 32–37].

How then do we apply the use of these measurements to our clinical practice? At the outset of our nutritional programme we assiduously measured all, or most, of the nutritional parameters, and indeed still do in the case of our clinical research programmes. Initially, decisions as to whether to institute nutritional support were based on the results of these measurements, particularly when doubt existed about the clinical diagnosis. As we gained more experience, however, we began to realise that one of the major roles of nutritional support is to prevent the development of protein calorie malnutrition. Consequently, our decisions as to whether to institute nutritional support are now influenced more by previous dietary history and the natural history of the primary disease process in respect of future nutritional intake than by measurements of nutritional parameters. In practical terms, we therefore currently place very little emphasis on the measurement of those parameters.

To become aware of protein calorie malnutrition is the most important key to improving the nutritional care of the hospitalised patient, so our recommendation to those in the field with relatively little experience would be, despite the various limitations, to take a clinical and dietary history, examine and weigh the patient, measure the midarm circumference and skinfold thicknesses, and measure the serum albumin and circulating lymphocyte count.

Monitoring treatment

In the last 3 years we have performed two controlled clinical trials of enteral nutritional products, and prospectively studied over 100 patients receiving parenteral nutrition as their only means of nutritional support. With the exception of the lymphocyte counts in the patients on parenteral nutrition and the transferrin levels following enteral nutrition [11], we have failed to show that a significant change has occurred in any of the other parameters in response to nutritional support. It should be pointed out, however, that our experience in respect of the skin testing data is not in agreement with that of a number of other groups [27, 29, 42].

In the light of our clinical experience, we would not necessarily advocate the routine monitoring of all the nutritional parameters listed in Table 3.1. Our overall aim is to provide effective nutritional support and thereby to place our patients in positive nitrogen balance. Nitrogen balances are computed very frequently (a minimum of three times a week) by carefully documenting intake and calculating output from values of urinary urea excretion (see Chapter 6). Patients should be monitored biochemically and haematologically at regular intervals to detect early onset of side-effects, so the serum albumin and lymphocyte count should be readily available as these will give the clinician some indirect guide as to the progress being made, although, as mentioned above, changes do not always occur. Caution should be taken before laying emphasis on any weight gains seen, particularly in patients being fed parenterally, as recent studies suggest that this is likely to be due to a gain in extracellular water rather than to changes in body fat or protein content [43].

PREDICTION OF POST-OPERATIVE MORBIDITY

In surgical circles, there is growing enthusiasm for vigorous nutritional support of malnourished patients about to undergo major surgery [44]. This argument is based on the premise that malnourished patients have more post-operative complications [45, 46] and even an increased risk of dying. Several groups are therefore investigating whether any reliance can be placed on the use of the nutritional parameters as a means of predicting patients at risk of developing post-operative complications. As Chapter 6 will show, there is very little hard evidence to show that pre-operative nutritional support offers any significant clinical benefit, and one of the reasons for this is that most studies of the subject have been concerned with unselected patients [47]. It should not come as a surprise that pre-operative nutritional support is without effect when administered to well-nourished patients, and the final answer to the question of whether pre-operative nutritional support has a significant beneficial effect can only be answered when preselected 'at risk' malnour-ished pre-operative surgical patients are prospectively ran-domised to receive their normal nutrient intake or formulated nutritional support.

WEIGHT LOSS

The addage that patients who have lost a lot of weight have a greater risk of dying was originally based upon figures showing a mortality rate following gastrectomy of 33.3% in patients who had lost more than 20% of body weight, compared to 3.5% [48] in patients with less than 20% weight loss. Prediction of post-operative complications and mortality based on weight loss is not nearly as simple as these figures imply, as the above findings suggesting that pre-operative weight loss is an important risk factor were made over 40 years ago, before antibiotics and modern chest physiotherapy. Analysis of this paper shows that nearly all deaths were related to chest infections, a complication that it would be reasonable to expect could be prevented today [44]. In fact there appears to be no recent data showing convincingly that there is a close relationship between the degree of weight loss prior to surgery and post-operative morbidity and mortality [49–51].

DELAYED HYPERSENSITIVITY SKIN TESTING

The findings that apparently malnourished patients have a high incidence of negative delayed hypersensitivity skin tests and that those patients with negative skin tests have an increased risk of post-operative sepsis [31, 52], lead to suggestions that delayed hypersensitivity skin testing can be used to predict post-operative sepsis and mortality. A later study confirmed that 'anergic' patients had a greater risk of developing post-operative complications and a higher mortality than those with positive responses to skin testing [53]. However, closer analysis of the two major studies [31, 53] shows that skin testing cannot be used as a single predictive test in the individual patient, as there were patients in both the positive and anergic groups who developed post-operative complications and died. In reality, therefore, the concept that a single pre-operative set of skin tests measuring delayed hypersensitivity can predict the long-term status of the patient is naive [54], and supporting evidence of this has been obtained by Irving and colleagues [50] who have found that skin testing was of no value in predicting post-operative sepsis or mortality.

MEASUREMENT OF PROTEIN STORES

Although hypoalbuminaemia has been claimed to accurately reflect malnutrition [41], a low pre-operative albumin concentration has proved to be a relatively insensitive predictor of post-operative morbidity [50, 51]. Transferrin [55] is a somewhat better predictor, but again its use as a single predictive test in an individual patient does not hold up. Concentrations of other serum proteins such as retinol-binding protein or thyroxin-binding prealbumin may prove more helpful, but have yet to be fully evaluated.

It has been suggested that estimation of skeletal muscle protein by measurement of arm muscle circumference predicts serious complications more reliably than measurement of weight, weight loss or serum albumin concentration [56]. As before, however, such claims do not bear close scrutiny, as in a larger survey 21%

of 184 patients with an arm muscle circumference greater than 85% of standard values developed post-operative complications [51].

The latest information is that a functional assessment of protein mass by grip strength dynamometry has a lower false-negative rate than the other tests and thus is a better screening test [51]. Thus 45% of 44 patients with impaired grip strengths developed complications compared with only 5% of 58 patients with normal values. These results are promising, but need confirmation because in the series of patients studied undergoing mainly cholecystectomy or gastroduodenal and colorectal operations there was an unusually high (24%) incidence of post-operative complications, defined only as an event that delayed the post-operative period in hospital by more than 14 days or resulted in death.

The only conclusion one can draw from these studies is that it is still a naive concept to believe that any single test of nutritional status is capable of reliably predicting post-operative outcome in an individual patient. As mentioned above, some groups are therefore now attempting to provide a prognostic nutritional index based on the use of several tests [38, 57, 58]. Further work is needed in this field, as it will only be possible to assess the clinical benefits of pre-operative nutritional support when 'at risk' patients can be reliably identified.

REFERENCES

1 Bristian B.R., Blackburn G.L., Hallowell E. & Heddle R. (1974) Protein status of general surgical patients. *J. Am. Med. Assoc.* **230**, 858.

2 Bristian B.R., Blackburn G.L., Vitale J., *et al* (1976) Prevalence of malnutrition in general medical patients. *J. Am. Med. Assoc.* **235**, 1597.

3 Hill G.L., Pickfort I., Young G.A., *et al* (1977) Malnutrition in surgical patients. An unrecognised problem. *Lancet* **i**, 689.

4 Leevy C.M., Cardi L., Frank O., *et al* (1965) Incidence and significance of hypovitaminaemia in a randomly selected municipal hospital population. *Am. J. Clin. Nutr.* **17**, 259.

5 Boolet A.J. & Owens S. (1973) Evaluation of nutritional status of selected hospitalised patients. *Am. J. Clin. Nutr.* **26**, 931.

6 Butterworth C.E. (1974) The skeleton in the hospital closet. *Nutr. Today* **9**, 4.

7 Walesby R.K., Goode A.W., Spinks J.J., *et al* (1979) Nutritional status of patients requiring cardiac surgery. *J. Thorac. Cardiovasc. Surg.* **77**, 570.

8 Ray K. & Dickerson J.W.T. (1979) Current practice in parenteral nutrition: results of a questionnaire. *J. Human. Nutr.* **33**, 288.

9   Goode A.W. (1981) The scientific basis of nutritional assessment. *Br. J. Anaesth.* **53**, 161.

10 Mueller C.B. & Thomas E.J. (1975) Nutritional needs of the normal adult. In *Manual of Surgical Nutrition*, eds. W.E. Ballinger, J.A. Collins, W.R. Drucker, S.J. Dudreck, R. Zeppa. W.B. Saunders, Philadelphia.

11 Jones B.J.M., Lees R., Andrews J. Frost P. & Silk D.B.A. (1983) Comparison of an elemental and polymeric enteral diet in patients with normal gastrointestinal function. *Gut* **24**, 78.

12 Keohane P.P., Jones B.J.M. & Silk D.B.A. (1981) Influence of lactose and *Cl. difficile* in the pathogenesis of enteral feeding associated diarrhoea. *J. Parent. Ent. Nutr.* **5**, 359.

13 James W.P.T. (1982) Assessment of nutritional status. *Med. Int.* **15**, 663.

14 Spiller R. & Silk D.B.A. (1982) Practical and experimental techniques to assess gastrointestinal tract function. In *Textbook of Enteral Nutrition*, eds. R.W. Luther and T.R. Sykes. Grune and Stratton, New York.

15 Fletcher R.F. (1962) The measurement of total body fat with skinfold calipers. *Clin. Sci.* **22**, 333.

16 Blackburn G.L. (1977) *Nutritional Support and Medical Practice*, eds. H.A. Schneider, C.E. Anderson and D.B. Coursin. Harper and Row, New York.

17 Collins J.P., McCarthy I.D. & Hull G.L. (1979) Assessment of protein nutrition in surgical patients—the value of anthropometrics. *Am. J. Clin. Nutr.* **32**, 1527.

18 Munro H. (1978) Biological limiting factors to parental amino acid feeding. In *Advances in Parental Nutrition*, ed. I.D.A. Johnston, p. 114. MTP Press, Lancaster.

19 Olusi S.A., McFarlane H., Osinkoya B.O. & Adesina H. (1975) Specific protein assays in protein calorie malnutrition. *Clin. Chim. Acta* **62**, 107.

20 Shetty P.S., Watrasiewicz K.E., Jung R.T. & James W.P.T. (1979) Rapid-turnover transport proteins: an index of subclinical protein energy malnutrition. *Lancet* ii, 230.

21 James W.P.T., Davies H.L. & Waterlow J.C. (1976) Nutritional aspects of plasma protein metabolism: the relevance of protein turnover rates during malnutrition and its remission in man. In *Plasma Protein Turnover*, eds. R. Bianchi, G. Mariani and A.S. McFarlane, p. 251. Macmillan, London.

22 Awai M. & Brown E.B. (1963) Studies of the metabolism of unlabelled human transferrin. *J. Lab. Clin. Med.* **61**, 363.

23 Ingenbleek Y., Can den Shriek H.G., De Nayer P., *et al* (1975) Albumin, transferrin and thyroxine binding prealbumin/retinol binding protein (TBA/RBP) complex in assessment of malnutrition. *Clin. Chim. Acta* **63**, 61.

24 Tavill A.S. & Kershenobick D. (1972) Regulation of transferrin synthesis. In *Protides of the Biological Fluids*, ed. H. Peeters, Proc., 19th Congress. Elsevier, Amsterdam.

25 Socolow E.L., Woehr K.A. & Purdy R.H. (1965) Preparation of ^{131}I labelled human serum prealbumin and its metabolism in normal and sick patients. *J. Clin. Invest.* **44**, 1600.

26 Peterson P.A. (1971) Demonstration in serum of two physiological forms of human retinol binding protein. *Eur. J. Clin. Invest.* **1**, 437.

27 Law D.K., Dudrick S.J. & Abdon N.I. (1973) Immunocompetence of patients with protein calorie malnutrition. Effects of nutritional repletion. *Ann. Int. Med.* **79**, 545.

28 Law D.K., Dudrick S.J. & Abdon N.I. (1974) The effect of dietary protein depletion on immunocompetence. The importance of nutritional repletion prior to immunologic induction. *Ann. Surg.* **179**, 168.

29 Spanier A.H., Pietsch J.B., Meakins J.L. *et al* (1976) Relationship between immune competence and nutrition. *Surg. Forum* **27**, 332.

30 Bristian B.R., Blackburn G.L., Scrimshaw N.S. & Flatt J.P. (1975) Cellular immunity in semi-starved states in hospitalised adults. *Am. J. Clin. Nutr.* **28**, 1148.

31 Pietsch J.B., Meakins J.L. & Maclean L.D. (1977) The delayed hypersensitivity response: application in clinical surgery. *Surgery* **82**, 349.

32 Johnson M.W., Maiback H.I. & Salmon S.W. (1971) Skin reactivity in patients with cancer. *New Engl. J. Med.* **284**, 1255.

33 Palmer D.L. & Reed W.P. (1974) Delayed hypersensitivity skin testing. II. Clinical correlates and anergy. *J. Infect. Dis.* **130**, 138.

34 Waldort D.S., Wilkens R.F. & Decker J.L. (1968) Impaired delayed hypersensitivity in an ageing population. Association with anti-nuclear reactivity and rheumatoid factor. *J. Am. Med. Assoc.* **203**, 831.

35 Saba T.M. (1975) Reticulo-endothelial system host defence after surgery and traumatic shock. *Circ. Shock* **2**, 91.

36 Pekarek R.S., Sandstead H.H., Jacob R.A. & Barcome D.F. (1979) Abnormal cellular immune responses during acquired zinc deficiency. *Am. J. Clin. Nutr.* **32**, 1466.

37 Chandra R.K. (1976) Iron and immunocompetence. *Nutr. Rev.* **34**, 129.

38 Buzby G.P., Mullen J.L., Matthews D.C., *et al* (1980) Prognostic nutritional index in gastrointestinal surgery. *Am. J. Surg.* **139**, 160.

39 Arullani A., Capello G., DeVittori, R., *et al* (1981) PCMI (proteo caloric malnutrition index): a nutritional index for surgical patients. *J. Parent. Ent. Nutr.* **5**, 352.

40 Klidjian A.M., Russell L. & Karran S.J. (1981) A malnutrition score for rapid nutritional assessment. In *Proceedings 1981 Surgical Research Society*.

41 Whitehead R., Coward W. & Lunn P.G. (1973) Serum albumin concentration and the onset of kwashiorkor. *Lancet* **ii**, 63.

42 Meakins J.L., Pietsch J.B., Bubewick O., *et al* (1977) Delayed hypersensitivity: indicator of acquired failure of host defences in sepsis and trauma. *Ann. Surg.* **186**, 241.

43 Yeung C.K., Smith R.C. & Hill G.L. (1979) Effect of an elemental diet on body composition. A comparison with intravenous nutrition. *Gastroenterology* **77**, 652.

44 Hill G.L. (1979) Do malnourished patients need nutritional therapy before major surgery? *Med. J. Austr.* **2**(9), 464–6.

45 Anonymous (1979) Parenteral nutrition before surgery. *Br. Med. J.* **2**, 1529.

46 Anonymous (1979) Malnutrition and cancer. *Br. Med. J.* **1**, 912.

47   Heatley R.V., Williams R.H.P. & Lewis M.H. (1979) Pre-operative intravenous feeding. A controlled trial. *Postgrad. Med. J.* **55**, 541.

48   Studley H.O. (1936) Percentage weight loss. A basic indicator of surgical risk in patients with chronic peptic ulcer. *J. Am. Med. Assoc.* **106**, 458.

49   Karran S.J., Cooper A.J., Foster K.J. & Kammerling R.M. (1980) Detection of dangerous pre-operative malnutrition. In *Proceedings 2nd European Congress of Parenteral and Enteral Nutrition*, p. 43.

50   Brown R., Hamid J., Patel N., *et al* (1980) The failure of delayed hypersensitivity skin testing to predict post-operative sepsis and mortality. In *Proceedings 2nd European Congress of Parenteral and Enteral Nutrition*, p. 37.

51   Klidjian A.M., Foster K.J., Kammerling R.M., *et al* (1980) Relation of anthropometric and dynomometric variables to serious post-operative complications. *Br. Med. J.* **281**, 899.

52   Maclean L.D., Meakins J.L., Taguchi K., *et al* (1975) Host resistance in sepsis and trauma. *Ann. Surg.* **182**, 207.

53   Johnson W.C., Ulrich F., Meguid M.M., *et al* (1979) Role of delayed hypersensitivity in predicting post-operative morbidity and mortality. *Am. J. Surg.* **137**, 536.

54   Wilson R.E. (1979) In discussion, role of delayed hypersensitivity in predicting post-operative morbidity and mortality. *Am. J. Surg.* **137**, 536.

55   Kaminski M.V., Fitzgerald M.J., *et al* (1977) Correlation of mortality with serum transferrin and anergy. *J. Parent. Ent. Nutr.* **1**, 27.

56   Kammerling R.M., Foster K.J. & Karran S.J. (1978) Protein depletion and recovery from surgical operation. *Br. J. Surg.* **65**, 365.

57   Nazari S., Comincioli V., Dionigi R., *et al* (1980) Cluster analysis of nutritional and immunological indicators for identification of increased susceptibility to surgical infections. In *Proceedings 2nd European Congress of Parenteral and Enteral Nutrition*, p 44.

58   Simms J.M. & Smith J.A.R. (1981) A prognostic index for surgical patients. *J. Parent. Ent. Nutr.* **5**, 353.

59   Bistian B.R., Blackburn G.L. & Sherman M. (1975) Therapeutic index of nutritional depletion in hospitalized patients. *Surg. Gynaec. Obstet.* **141**, 152.

Chapter 4
Indications for
Nutritional Support

It is usually traditional to catagorise those clinical conditions that may be frequently associated with protein calorie malnutrition and to imply that patients with these conditions are those likely to require nutritional support. Table 4.1, for example, summarises such a list of conditions. In the light of our recent experience such an approach seems to be a gross over-simplification of the problems that arise when deciding whether or not to institute nutritional support. This is not least of all because, as one's experience of clinical nutrition in hospital medicine broadens, almost all medical or surgical conditions *can* be accompanied by protein calorie malnutrition.

The indications for the provision of nutritional support as defined in the Central Middlesex Hospital are summarised in Table 4.2. It has always been our policy to provide this support to the obviously and severely malnourished patient (severe weight loss, marked muscle wasting and hypoproteinaemic oedema).

If there is doubt about the clinical diagnosis, but a dietary history shows impaired nutrient intake for more than one week and the nutritional parameters are suggestive of protein calorie malnutrition, then consideration will be given to providing nutritional support.

We now quite often provide nutritional support to a third group of patients who, on admission, may be reasonably well nourished. This is a group of patients who we think will develop malnutrition if we withhold nutritional support, and includes those undergoing neurosurgery or those with neurologically based disorders such as strokes, bulbar palsies or motorneurone disease. The inclusion of such patients in our nutritional programme has come about as a result of the knowledge we have gained of the natural history of disorders not necessarily familiar to us as gastroenterologists, and our acknowledgement that one of the important functions of nutritional support is to prevent protein calorie malnutrition from developing in hospital in-patients.

Our efforts to provide nutritional support to neurosurgical patients have been rewarded by easier mobilisation in the

Table 4.1 Disease states associated with protein calorie malnutrition.

Pre- and post-operative patients

Cancer

Inflammatory bowel disease

Pancreatitis

Severe trauma

Burns

Sepsis

Liver failure

Renal failure

Table 4.2 Indications for nutritional support.

---

1 Obvious gross malnutrition: albumin < 30 g/l; marked weight loss; muscle wasting; oedema
2 Nutritional parameters suggestive of protein calorie malnutrition—dietary history shows impaired nutrient intake for one week or more
3 Medical and surgical disorders likely to result in protein calorie malnutrition if nutritional support withheld

---

post-operative period, virtual disappearance of bed sores and shorter in-patient stay. A controlled clinical trial is in progress in Nottingham to determine whether nutritional support affords advantages in the management of elderly patients admitted to the orthopaedic wards with fractures. It seems reasonable to suppose that similar findings will arise from this study.

Notwithstanding our rather generalised approach to the indications for nutritional support, certain specific indications do exist; for example, in burns patients and those with enterocutaneous fistulae. In addition, considerable interest has surrounded the use of nutritional support in pre- and post-operative states, in inflammatory bowel disease as well as an adjunct to cancer therapy. The ensuing paragraphs discuss some of the areas of interest in these fields. The applications of nutritional support to the areas of liver disease and renal failure are covered later (see Chapters 9, 10).

PRE-OPERATIVE NUTRITIONAL SUPPORT

As outlined in the previous chapter, there is growing enthusiasm for vigorous nutritional support for malnourished patients about to undergo major surgery. Despite this, there is extremely little evidence available to show clinical benefits. One of the major reasons for this is that unselected patients have been included in the clinical trials of pre-operative nutrition, and possible conclusions that might have been drawn from the trials have been obscured as a result of the inclusion of normally nourished patients. The inclusion of such patients in turn is part due to the difficulties that exist in not only diagnosing protein calorie malnutrition, but also in defining simple measurements that can accurately predict post-operative morbidity and mortality.

Other problems that make this area so confusing include definitions of 'major abdominal operations'. Some authors, for example, include patients in their studies who are undergoing elective cholecystectomy—in reasonable hands hardly a major abdominal procedure. Difficulties arise in interpreting the term 'post-operative complication', and these seem to vary from 'wound infections' [1], to delay in post-operative hospital stay [2]. Furthermore, the picture is often confused by the inclusion in many series of cancer patients, some of whom in their own right might be expected to develop a higher incidence of post-operative complications than non-cancer patients. Finally, and most importantly, it must be appreciated that different surgeons are capable of producing different incidences of post-operative complications, e.g. anastomotic leaks following anterior resection of the colon [3]. Thus, it does not necessarily follow that the possible benefits of pre-operative nutritional support occurring from one centre will be applicable to others.

Notwithstanding these problems, trials have been published suggesting benefits of pre-operative nutritional support. Bojanowicz [4] showed that patients undergoing colonic surgery had a significantly lower incidence of post-operative wound infection if they received a course of enteral nutrition in the pre-operative period. No attempts were made, however, to categorise the patients according to nutritional status. In a widely quoted study, Heatley and colleagues [1] purported to show an advantage of pre-operative parenteral nutrition in patients with gastric or oesophageal cancer in respect of the incidence of wound infection, irrespective of whether the serum albumin was below 35 g/l or not. The study is open to criticism, however, as the control and treatment groups were not equally matched for nitrogen losses, all those undergoing oesophageal anastamosis received post-operative parenteral nutrition, and no attempt was made to monitor intakes of a liquidised diet administered to both groups in the pre-operative period. A sounder study has recently been performed by Mueller and colleagues [5], who in a larger series of patients have shown that the incidence of major complications and mortality in patients undergoing surgery for cancer of the gastrointestinal tract were significantly reduced by 10 days pre-operative parenteral nutrition. In contrast to these two studies [1, 5], no clear-cut benefit of pre-operative parenteral nutrition was seen by Simms and colleagues [6] in other patients undergoing major gastric or oesophageal resection for malignant disease.

There is thus remarkably little evidence upon which to base any serious claims that routine pre-operative nutritional support confers clinically significant benefits in respect of post-operative outcome. How then is the clinician best advised about the nutritional care of his patient about to undergo surgery? On present evidence there would appear to be no justification for providing routine pre-operative nutritional support of the well-nourished patient. As some of the above data do indicate benefits, despite the inclusion of well-nourished patients, it seems reasonable to advise pre-operative nutritional support to the obviously malnourished patient about to undergo major surgery. If more than 10% of previous body weight has been lost, the albumin is less than 35 g/l, or the lymphocyte count less than 1200/mm^3, nutritional support via the enteral or parenteral route for 7–10 days is likely to improve the post-operative outlook. The number of patients will not be very large, and in the Leeds group only 3–4% of patients were considered to suffer from protein calorie malnutrition of a degree that it was considered beneficial to provide pre-operative nutritional support [7].

POST-OPERATIVE NUTRITIONAL SUPPORT

Arguments have been put forward that certain groups of patients should receive nutritional support routinely in the post-operative period. Confusion surrounds this subject, just as it does with pre-operative nutrition, mainly on account of the fact that so many apparently well-nourished patients have been included in the various series.

Early post-operative total parenteral nutrition significantly reduced the incidence of post-operative complications following abdominoperineal resection of the colon [8], but not in major gastric or gastro-oesophageal resections for malignant disease [6]. Early post-operative fine needle catheter jejunostomy feeding after major gastrointestinal surgery had no effect on the post-operative complication rate [9], although marginal benefits occurred in respect of length of hospital stay when an elemental diet was instilled into the upper small intestine during the first week after surgery [10]. It has now been established that the routine use of parenteral nutrition following total cystectomy, when groups of patients are considered, cannot be justified [11].

These few examples serve to illustrate the difficulties surrounding the use of *routine* nutritional support in the post-operative period. In our unit we have no absolute policy defined for post-operative nutrition. In the severely malnourished patient coming to elective surgery, pre-operative nutritional support is instituted prior to operation. If the patient is haemodynamically and electrolytically stable post-operatively, nutritional support is continued in the immediate post-operative period, usually via the parenteral route. If haemodynamic and electrolyte problems arise in the immediate post-operative period, these are usually corrected before nutritional support is continued. If patients are not severely malnourished then decisions to implement post-operative nutrition are based upon the clinical course. If it is apparent that post-operative recovery is likely to be delayed we institute nutritional support sooner rather than later, according to our belief that one of its major functions is to prevent the onset of significant protein calorie malnutrition.

NUTRITION AND CANCER

The area of nutrition in cancer has stimulated a great deal of interest of late [12], and in America the National Cancer Institute has recently been persuaded to spend more time on studying the cause and treatment of malnutrition in patients with cancer [12]. Interest arises in part from the claims that nutritional support improves the clinical outcome of treatment—whether by resection of the tumour, by chemotherapy or by radiotherapy [12]. As will be shown, the first wave of published reports were based largely upon uncontrolled and anecdotal data; controlled trials and the fashionable backlash in opinion are beginning to make an appearance.

Effect of nutritional support on tumour growth

One important question that continues to be raised is whether improved nutritional status leads to increased tumour growth. The only objective studies aimed at answering this question have been carried out in tumour-bearing animals, and even in such models results are conflicting. In two of three reports parenteral nutrition did not increase the relative tumour weight or size [14, 15], in one report tumour growth was stimulated [16]. It should be borne in mind, though, that the animal tumours may account for up to 30% of the total body weight, whereas patients with metastatic cancer rarely have a tumour burden of more than 10% of their weight, and it is very rare for a patient to have an explosive tumour growth such as is seen in these animals [17]. It follows, therefore, that it is probably futile to extrapolate any evidence from rodent studies to man [12].

It would be expected, however, that there should be some increased growth of residual tumour in patients as a result of improved nutrition since tumour cells, like host cells, have a dependency on good nutrition. Moreover, there are grounds for believing that improved nutrition may be therapeutically useful since actively dividing cells are more likely to be sensitive to radiation or chemotherapy than slowly dividing cells, and this is borne out by preliminary results of animal studies [18, 19]. On balance, therefore, it is unlikely that the provision of nutritional support will have any deleterious effect on primary tumour therapy. However, more objective data is needed before actual claims can be made that nutritional support is associated with decreased radiation or chemotherapy toxicity and/or improved clinical response and survival.

Effectiveness of nutritional support on nutritional status of cancer patients

The basal metabolic rate of cancer patients is higher than that of non-cancerous controls [20], energy expenditure in excess of intake has been reported [21] and obviously contributes to weight loss. The energy required to maintain weight in the cancer patient therefore exceeds the normal requirement, a factor that has to be considered when formulating the nutritional programme for the cancer patient. The needs for specific nutrients such as ascorbic acid [22], thiamine [23] and vitamin A [24] may also be high compared with non-cancerous patients.

As in other areas, most of the documented effects of nutritional support in cancer patients are mainly concerned with the effects of parenteral rather than enteral nutrition. The general consensus of recent studies is that nutritional status can be improved in the cancer patient, but often less effectively than in equivalent malnourished, non-cancer-bearing groups [25]. Much of the data pertaining to weight gain is difficult to interpret since significant proportions of the gains during parenteral nutrition may be due to fluid retention [26], and although cancer-bearing patients appear able to create fat equally as well as their malnourished non-cancer-bearing controls [27], protein stores may not be so efficiently repleted [28].

Nutritional support in specific areas

Pre- and post-operative nutritional support

The difficulties in defining the benefits of pre and post-operative nutrition discussed above particularly apply to cancer patients. In the few available properly controlled studies of pre-operative nutrition, a significant proportion of cancer patients were included [1, 4, 5, 8]. Future studies, if confined to properly defined malnourished and 'at risk' patients, will almost certainly show that pre- and post-operative nutritional support has a role as an adjunct to surgical treatment of the cancer patient.

As an adjunct to palliative therapy

Results of available studies indicate that nutritional support has little or no influence on survival [29] or in the ability of patients to tolerate a therapeutic regime [30]. Indeed, in one study there was a suggestion that parenteral nutrition decreased survival in patients with metastatic colorectal cancer treated with 5FU and methyl CCNU [31].

As an adjunct to chemotherapy

It is difficult to make recommendations about the role of nutritional support as an adjunct to chemotherapy because so few trials have been performed. Promising results of parenteral nutrition in acute leukaemias have been reported both in respect of numbers of remissions and survival [32], it is not clear, though, why nutritional support was administered by the parenteral rather than enteral route. In contrast, parenteral nutrition did not improve the quantity of drugs administered to patients receiving aggressive therapy for diffuse histiocytic lymphoma [33], nor was the tolerance to therapy, as determined by haematological toxicity, improved. Finally, it does not seem that non-operative treatment of oat cell carcinoma of the lung is influenced in any major clinically significant way by nutritional support [34, 35].

Nutritional support during or following radiotherapy

The clinical effects of ionising radiation to various portions of the alimentary tract have been reviewed in detail [36] and it is well acknowledged that radiotherapy to the head and neck, often in conjunction with surgery, or to the abdomen, may result in nutritional problems related to difficulties in ingesting, chewing, swallowing or absorbing food. There are no specific indications for nutritional support in these circumstances, and the decision to institute nutritional support should be based upon the nutritional status of the patient as well as on the natural history of the different complications.

Conclusions

It follows from the above discussion that the exact roles of nutritional support in cancer have not yet been properly defined. Controlled trials are currently under way in a number of major centres, so there will probably be more data available for critical evaluation in the near future. At present, it would seem that patients who will respond to treatment should not be allowed to go malnourished. Conversely, patients who will not respond should not be maintained on unnecessary nutritional support.

NUTRITIONAL SUPPORT IN INFLAMMATORY BOWEL DISEASE

There is a large and generally unspectacular literature on the influences that nutritional support has had on the short- as well as long-term management of inflammatory bowel disease. With a few exceptions, it is almost impossible to critically evaluate the results because of the absence of control groups.

Patients with inflammatory bowel disease constitute a population that are often malnourished [37]. Many of the reports have therefore been concerned with improvements achieved in nutritional status, usually in combination with bowel rest and, at the same time, the authors have attempted to draw conclusions about patient outcome, particularly in relationship to the avoidance of surgical intervention [38–40]. Despite the drawbacks of many of the studies, it must be admitted that there are problems inherent in trial design of patients with inflammatory bowel disease, not only because of the difficulties that occur in reaching a precise diagnosis, but also because of differences that exist in duration, extent and severity of the disease, all of which may affect the response to therapy.

Four important conclusions can be drawn from the information available.

1 Nutritional support, administered either by the enteral or parenteral route, in combination with medical therapy, frequently results in an improvement of the nutritional status of patients with inflammatory bowel disease (IBD) [37–44]. There

appears no reason, however, to advocate the use of the parenteral rather than enteral route of administration, and not one scrap of clinical evidence to advocate the use of the so-called chemically defined elemental diets over the related low-residue polymeric diets. Moreover, the evidence that a low-residue nutritionally formulated diet is in any way superior to a diet containing normal or increased amounts of residue is also lacking.

2   The immediate outcome of patients with colitis, due either to Crohn's disease or ulcerative colitis, is uninfluenced by parenteral nutrition [44], which cannot therefore be considered as a primary therapy.

3   Decisions as to whether to recommend surgery in malnourished patients with small intestinal Crohn's disease should not be made until efforts have been made to improve the nutritional status of these patients. This is because there is a strong suggestion from uncontrolled studies that if an early decision to proceed to surgery is made while the patient is still malnourished, surgery may be rendered unnecessary in a significant proportion of patients by subsequent nutritional support [38–42].

4   Abnormal growth patterns in children with Crohn's disease may be restored by means of short or long term enteral nutrition using both elemental and polymeric diets in combination with medical therapy [45, 46].

ENTEROCUTANEOUS FISTULAE

Few would disagree that the introduction of nutritional support has had a major impact on the mortality of patients with enterocutaneous fistulae. Overall mortality before the realisation of the importance of nutritional support was in the region of 40–45% [47, 48], and as high as 60% in patients considered malnourished [47]. Since the introduction of nutritional support [49], mortality has fallen to between 9 and 34% [50–52].

Despite the undoubted impact that nutritional support has had on fistulae mortality and healing, the mechanism of its action is far from understood, and controversy exists as to whether nutritional support with bowel rest (i.e. parenteral nutrition) is superior to enteral nutrition using an elemental diet, which has been shown to marginally reduce ileostomy output as well as the volume of ileal fistula effluent [53, 54]. Yet again there are no controlled clinical trials to answer this point.

In the management of the fistulae, basic surgical principles must be adhered to. Thus, if radiological studies show obstruction distal to the fistula, neither parenteral or enteral nutrition is likely to increase the chances of the fistula closing [55], and in these cases the best that these can hope to achieve is improvement of nutritional status prior to surgery.

In the clinical experience of the author, attempts to close enterocutaneous fistulae in patients with Crohn's disease usually fail when nutritional support is provided via the enteral route, and as long as there is no distal obstruction or underlying malignancy, closure of other fistulae is also achieved quicker with parenteral, rather than enteral, nutrition.

ACUTE PANCREATITIS

Patients with acute pancreatitis constitute a further group of patients who, under certain circumstances, require nutritional support. 70–80% of patients seem to run a limiting course and, after the abdominal pain and ileus, if present, resolve introduction of oral feeding is possible, usually within about five days or so. These patients do not require nutritional support.

In about a fifth of cases [56], the pancreatitis persists for longer, or the patients develop haemorrhage or post-necrotic pancreatitis, or the pancreatitis is complicated by an abscess or pseudocyst function. In these, some form of nutritional support is mandatory, particularly since these patients are often hypermetabolic with nitrogen losses in excess of 15 g a day.

It is traditional teaching that 'resting' the gastrointestinal tract is helpful in allowing the inflammatory process to subside [56]. Although we have never been over-impressed with these claims, many of the patients have a localised ileus which makes nutritional support via the enteral route impractical. Moreover since a significant proportion may require surgery in one form or another, we are happy to institute parenteral nutrition. We agree with others [57] that few problems arise with parenteral nutrition in these patients, either with hyperglycaemia (insulin supplements may be required) or with use of a triglyceride-based energy source.

In our unit we believe that severe pancreatitis is definitely one of the situations in which the patients benefit from nutritional support.

SEVERE BURNS

The patient with severe burns has the most accelerated rate of tissue breakdown associated with any disease process. Without adequate nutritional support an adult with 40% full thickness burns will lose 30% of his body weight in less than three weeks and will almost certainly die [58]. All the modern techniques of fluid resuscitation and skin grafting will not alter this prognosis without adequate nutritional support [59].

The accelerated rates of tissue breakdown occur on account of prodigious increases in the basal metabolic rate (BMR). BMR increases in a linear manner with increased burn size up to 40–50% of the total body surface and thereafter reaches a plateau [60], suggesting that patients with large burns attain maximum or near maximum levels of heat production (BMR 60–80% increased).

One of the problems that arises when considering nutritional support in the burn patient is the calculation of requirements. Guidelines have been developed from measurements made of metabolic rates and careful estimates of urinary and burn exudate nitrogen, and the protein and calorie requirements of the average patient can be predicted from the formula devised by Sutherland [61]. This formula takes into account the patient's weight, the size of the burn, and the different requirements of children and adults.

Whenever possible nutritional support should be provided by the enteral rather than parenteral route. Up to 4000 kcal/day can usually be provided via this route [59]. The indications for parenteral nutrition in the burned patient have been summarised by Davenport [59] as:

1 Those patients with disturbed gastrointestinal function.
2 Those patients unable to tolerate nasogastric feeding on account of severe facial or nasal burns.
3 Those patients who are unable to take sufficient nutrition down the nasogastric tube who require 'topping up' with additional intravenous feeding.

One of the greatest disadvantages of nasogastric feeding is associated with the frequent dressings and several operations that may be required during the course of their illness; each anaesthetic, even using the most modern techniques, requires an empty stomach before induction and this entails a period of starvation before, during and after treatment. In the future it is hoped that this problem can be overcome by the use of the more refined techniques of nasojejunal feeding.

REFERENCES

1 Heatley R.V., Williams R.H.P. & Lewis M.H. (1979) Pre-operative intravenous feeding—a controlled trial. *Postgrad. Med. J.* **55,** 541.
2 Klidjian A.M., Foster K.J. & Kammerling R.M. (1980) Relation of

anthropometric and dynamometric variables to serious post-operative complications. *Br. Med. J.* **281**, 899.

3   Fielding L.P., Stewart-Brown S. & Dudley H.A.F. (1978) Surgeon-related variables and the clinical trial. *Lancet* **ii**, 778.

4   Bojanowicz K. (1977) Anwendung der chemisch definierten Diät bei und nach Kolon Karzinom-Operationen. *Z. Ernährungswissenschaft.* suppl 20, 14.

5   Mueller J.M., Rose R., Arndt M. & Pichlmaier H. (1981) The value of pre-operative nutritional support in cancer surgery. *J. Parent. Ent. Nutr.* **5**, 357.

6   Simms J.M., Oliver E. & Smith J.A.R. (1980) A study of total parenteral nutrition (TPN) in major gastric and oesophageal resection for neoplasia. In *Proceedings 2nd European Congress on Parenteral and Enteral Nutrition*, p 37.

7   Hill G.L. (1979) Do malnourished patients need nutritional therapy before major surgery? *Med. J. Aust.* **2**(9), 464.

8   Collins J.P., Oxby C.B. & Hill G.L. (1978) Intravenous amino acids and intravenous hyperalimentation as protein-sparing therapy after major surgery. A controlled clinical trial. *Lancet* **i**, 788.

9   Yeung C.K., Young G.A., Hachett A.F. & Hill G.L. (1979) Fine needle catheter jejunostomy—an assessment of a new method of nutritional support after major gastro-intestinal surgery. *Br. J. Surg.* **66**, 733.

10 Sagar S., Harland R. & Shield R. (1979) Early post-operative feeding with elemental diet. *Br. Med. J.* **1**, 293.

11 Simms J.M. & Smith J.A.R. (1981) Intravenous feeding after total cystectomy—a controlled trial. In *Proceedings 3rd European Congress on Parenteral and Enteral Nutrition*, p 69.

12 Anonymous (1979) Malnutrition and cancer. *Br. Med. J.* **1**, 912.

13 Greenberg D.S. (1978) Washington Report. The Cancer Institute on the griddle. *New Engl. J. Med.* **299**, 207.

14 Daly J.M., Copeland E.M., Quinn E. & Dudrick S.J. (1976) Relationship of protein nutrition to tumour growth and host immunocompetence. *Surg. Forum* **27**, 113.

15 Steiger E., Oram-Smith J., Miller E., *et al* (1975) Effects of nutrition on tumour growth and tolerance to chemotherapy. *J. Surg. Res.* **18**, 455.

16 Cameron J.L. & Parlat W.A. (1976) Stimulation of growth of a transplantable hepatoma in rats by parenteral nutrition. *J. Nat. Cancer Inst.* **56**, 597.

17 Shils M.E. (1979) Nutrition and the cancer patient. *Nutrition and Cancer* **1**, 9.

18 Cameron J.L. & Rogers W. (1977) Total intravenous hyperalimentation and hydroxy urea chemotherapy in hepatoma bearing. *J. Surg. Res.* **23**, 279.

19 Reynolds H.M., Daly J.M., Copeland E.M. & Dudrick S.J. (1978) Effects of nutritional repletion on host and tumour responses to chemotherapy. *Fed. Proc.* **37**, 261.

20 Dickerson J.W.T. (1981) The role of enteral nutrition in malignant disease. *Acta Chir. Scand.* Suppl 507, 422.

21 Warnold I., Lundholm K. & Schersten T. (1978) Energy balance and body composition in cancer patients. *Cancer Res.* **38**, 1801.

22 Dickerson J.W.T. & Basu T.K. (1977) Specific vitamin deficiencies

and their significance in patients with cancer and receiving chemotherapy. In *Nutrition and Cancer*, ed. M. Winick, p 95. John Wiley, Chichester.

23 Aksoy M., Basu T.K. Brient J. & Dickerson J.W.T. (1983) Thiamine status of patients treated with drug combinations containing 5-fluorouracil. *Eur. J. Cancer* (in press).

24 Soukop M., VicKie J.G. & Calman K.C. (1978) Vitamin A status and chemotherapeutic response. In *Current Chemotherapy Proceedings of the International Congress of Chemotherapy*, p 1269.

25 Brennan M.F. (1981) Total parenteral nutrition in the management of the cancer patient. *Acta Chir. Scand.* Suppl 507, 428.

26 Yeung C.K., Smith R.C. & Hill G.L. (1979) Effect of an elemental diet on body composition. A comparison with intravenous nutrition. *Gastroenterology* 77, 652.

27 Nixon D., Rudman D., Heymsfield S., *et al* (1978) Response to nutritional support in cachetic patients. *Am. Assoc. Cancer Res.* (abstract), 698.

28 Brennan M.F. & Burt M.E. (1980) Nitrogen metabolism in cancer. *Cancer Treatment Report* (in press).

29 Solassol C., Joyenz H. & Dubois J.B. (1979) Total parenteral nutrition (TPN) with complete nutritive mixtures. An artificial gut in cancer patients. *Nutr. Cancer* 1, 13.

30 Valerio D., Overett M.T., Malcolm A. & Blackburn G.L. (1978) Nutritional support for cancer patients receiving abdominal and pelvin radiotherapy. A randomised, prospective clinical experiment of intravenous vs oral feeding. *Surg. Forum* 29, 145.

31 Nixon D., Kutner M.H., Ansley J., *et al.* (1980) Survival with and without hyperalimentation. *Cancer Treatment Report* (in press).

32 Coquin J.Y., Naraninchi D., Gastant J.A. & Carcassone Y. (1981) Influence of parenteral nutrition (PM) on chemotherapy and survival of acute leukaemias (AL). In *Proceedings 3rd European Congress on Parenteral and Enteral Nutrition*, p 68.

33 Popp M.B., Fischer R.I., Simon R.M. & Brennan M.F. (1981) A prospective randomised study of adjuvant parenteral nutrition in the treatment of diffuse lymphoma. 1. Effect on drug tolerance. *Cancer Treatment Report* (in press).

34 Lanzotti V., Copeland E.M., Bhuchar V., *et al* (1980) A randomised trial of total parenteral nutrition (TPM) with chemotherapy for non-oat cell cancer (MCCLC) *American Society of Clinical Oncology* (abstract), C-277.

35 Serrou B. & Cupissol B. (1980) Adjunct effect of parenteral intravenous nutrition (PIVM) depends on the tumour sensitivity to chemotherapy. *American Society of Clinical Oncology* (abstract), C-157.

36 Donaldson S. (1977) Nutritional consequences of radiotherapy. *Cancer Res.* 37, 2407.

37 Driscoll R.H. & Rosenberg I.H. (1978) Total parenteral nutrition in inflammatory bowel disease. *Med. Clin. N. Am.* 62, 185.

38 Fischer J.E., Foster G.S., Abel R.M., *et al* (1973) Hyperalimentation as primary therapy for inflammatory bowel disease. *Am. J. Surg.* 125, 165.

39 Vogel C.M., Corwin T.R. & Bane A.E. (1974) Intravenous hyperali-

mentation in the treatment of inflammatory diseases of the bowel. *Arch. Surg.* **108**, 460.

40 Reilly J., Ryan J.A., Strole W. & Fischer J.E. (1976) Hyper-alimentation in inflammatory bowel disease. *Am. J. Surg.* **131**, 192.

41 Rocchio M.A., Cha C.J.M., Haas K.F. & Randall H.T. (1974) Use of chemically defined diets in the management of patients with acute inflammatory bowel disease. *Am. J. Surg.* **127**, 469.

42 Voitk A.J., Echave V., Feller J.H., *et al* (1973) Experience with elemental diet in the treatment of inflammatory bowel disease. *Arch. Surg.* **107**, 329.

43 O'Marain C., Segal A.W. & Levi A.J. (1980) Elemental diets in the treatment of Crohn's disease. *Gut* **21**, A468.

44 Dickinson R.J., Ashton M.G., Axon A.T.R., *et al* (1980) Controlled trial of intravenous hyperalimentation and total bowel rest as an adjunct to the routine therapy of acute colitis. *Gastroenterology* **79**, 1199.

45 Morin C.L., Roulet M., Roy C.C. & Weber A. (1980) Continuous elemental enteral alimentation in children with Crohn's disease and growth failure. *Gastroenterology* **79**, 1205.

46 Kirschner B.S., Klich J.R. & Kalman S.S. (1981) Reversal of growth retardation in Crohn's disease with therapy emphasising oral nutritional restitution. *Gastroenterology* **80**, 10.

47 Edmunds L.H., Williams G.M. & Welch C.E. (1960) External fistulas arising from the gastrointestinal tract. *Ann. Surg.* **152**, 445.

48 Chapman R., Foran R. & Dunphy J.E. (1964) Management of intestinal fistulas. *Am. J. Surg.* **108**, 157.

49 Anonymous (1979) Nutritional management of enterocutaneous fistulas. *Lancet* **ii**, 507.

50 Sheldon G.F., Gardiner B.N., Way L.W. & Dunphy J.E. (1971) Management of gastrointestinal fistulas. *Surg. Gynaecol. Obstet.* **133**, 385.

51 Dietal M. (1976) Nutritional management of external gastrointestinal fistulas. *Can. J. Surg.* **19**, 505.

52 Thomas R.J.S. & Rosalion A. (1978) The use of parenteral nutrition in the management of external gastrointestinal tract fistulae. *Aust. NZ J. Surg.* **48**, 535.

53 Hill G.L., Mair W.S.J., Edwards J.P., *et al.* (1975) Effect of a chemically defined liquid elemental diet on composition and volume of ileal fistula drainage. *Gastroenterology* **68**, 676.

54 Hill G.L., Mair W.S.J., Edwards J.P. & Goligher J.C. (1976) Decreased trypsin and bile acids in ileal fistula drainage during the administration of a chemically defined liquid elemental diet. *Br. J. Surg.* **63**, 133.

55 Reilly J. (1976) Inflammatory bowel disease. In *Total Parenteral Nutrition*, ed. J.E. Fischer, p. 187. Little Brown, Boston.

56 Gliedman M.L., Boboki H. & Rosen R.G. (1970) Acute pancreatitis. *Current Problems in Surgery*, pp. 1–52.

57 Warshaw A.L., Imbembo A.L., Civetta J.M. & Daggett W.M. (1974) Surgical intervention in acute necrotising pancreatitis. *Am. J. Surg.* **127**, 4821.

58 Abbott W.M. (1976) Indications for parenteral nutrition. In *Total Parenteral Nutrition*, ed. J.E. Fischer, p. 1. Little Brown, Boston.

59 Davenport P.J. (1979) Nutritional support in severe burns. *Res. Clin. Forums* **1**, 79.

60 Wilmore D.W. & Pruitt B.A. (1976) Parenteral nutrition in burn patients. In *Total Parenteral Nutrition*, ed. J.E. Fischer, p. 231. Little Brown, Boston.

61 Sutherland A.B. (1976) Nitrogen balance and nutritional requirements in the burn patient: a reappraisal. *Burns* **2**, 238.

Chapter 5
Metabolic Responses to Starvation and Injury

Over 50 years ago, Cuthbertson first showed that there was a substantial mobilisation of protein in response to bone injury [1]. He envisaged that the increased output of urinary nitrogen represented a primitive reflex to supply energy needed for survival when an adequate fuel supply could not be ingested.

This demonstration that substantial protein losses occur in response to trauma signalled the beginning of a systematic analysis of the body's metabolic response to injury and surgery that still continues today.

The overall aim of nutritional support is to satisfy the nutritional requirements of the patient in order to ensure the maximum chances of survival when appropriate amounts of food cannot be ingested. The nutritional requirements can only be assessed if the clinician has some background knowledge of the metabolic changes that occur in response to not only injury but also starvation. Unfortunately the mass of data that has accumulated is often confusing, and those wanting practical help may be somewhat daunted by the fine detailed arguments put forward by some authors. This chapter, therefore, reviews some of the metabolic changes that occur in response to starvation and injury in a way that hopefully will simplify the subject matter and enable the clinician to grasp the basic points to a degree that enables him to formulate nutritional regimes that suit the requirements of different types of malnourished patients.

Several factors contribute to the malnutrition seen in hospitalised patients. In our experience probably the commonest is an inadequate intake of nutrients prior to admission due to the underlying disease process (e.g. mechanical dysphagia due to a carcinoma of the oesophagus). In two recent controlled trials our patients had received an inadequate diet for a mean period of between 2 and 3 weeks before enteral nutrition was instituted [2, 3]. Metabolically the changes that occur in these patients are synonymous with 'starvation'. The second major factor contributing to malnutrition is the 'injury' sustained, and in this context the term 'injury' includes trauma, surgery, sepsis and burns. At the outset it should be appreciated that the metabolic responses to starvation and injury are quite different, and form the basis of the contrasting nutritional requirements of the two types of patient.

It will also follow on from the discussion of the metabolic responses to starvation and injury that the starved patient can also sustain injury in hospital—for example, the starved patient with gastric or oesophageal cancer undergoing surgery. In terms of the metabolic changes that occur, a mixed picture emerges which results in changes occurring in the nutritional requirements during the course of the illness.

STARVATION   (Table 5.2)

The metabolic changes that occur in response to starvation are all geared to reducing the losses of body constituents to a minimum

Table 5.1   Fuel composition of normal man (after [5]).

Fuel	kg	Calories	Total
Tissues			
Fat (adipose triglyceride)	15	141 000	
Protein (mainly muscle)	6	24 000	165 900
Glycogen (muscle)	0.15	600	
Glycogen (liver)	0.075	300	
Circulating fuels			
Glucose (extracellular fluid)	0.020	80	
Plasma free fatty acids	0.0003	3	113
Triglycerides	0.003	30	

Table 5.2   Metabolic response to starvation (data from [4]).

Metabolic rate	Reduced
Hormonal changes	(a) Early small increases in catecholamines, glucagon, cortisol, growth hormone. Then slow fall. (b) Insulin decreased.
Energy production	Protein and fat early on then almost all from fat.
Nitrogen	Losses reduced
Weight loss	Slow
Water and sodium	Initial loss. Late retention

[4]. The first response is a small rise in catecholamines and glucagon which act to mobilise the glycogen stored in muscle and liver [5]. Glycogen is converted to the energy-producing substrate glucose. As can be seen in Table 5.1, the potential energy production from glycogen and circulating glucose is minute when compared with that from fat and protein. In practical terms the reserves are only sufficient for 24–48 hours [6].

Early on in starvation there is a rapid fall in weight, due to losses of water and sodium [7] not other essential body consti-tuents. At the same time two important hormonal changes occur. Circulating insulin levels fall and glucagon levels rise [7]. The subtle changes produced in the circulating insulin-glucagon ratio result in release of adipose triglycerides and breakdown of muscle protein. Branched-chain amino acids are oxidised by muscle, thereby acting on energy substrates [8]. Alanine formed in muscle tissue by transamination of pyruvate denied from glucose breakdown is then transported to the liver, where alanine acts as an energy substrate by means of its conversion to glucose (gluconeogenesis). The essential amino acids not utilised as an energy source in muscle enter the extracellular amino acid pool and are utilised by the liver for synthesis of albumin and other essential tissue proteins.

The triglycerides released from adipose tissue are hydrolysed to free fatty acids, which act as powerful energy substrates, either by direct conversion to acetyl CoA, or by final conversion to CoA derivates of the ketone bodies [8].

There exists a delicate relationship between the relative contribution of protein and triglyceride toward energy produc-tion. Initially relatively high proportions of energy arise from the breakdown of protein, and it has been estimated that if protein breakdown to provide a glucose energy source were to continue at initial rates found in acute starvation, death would occur by the tenth day [9]. Fortunately, as time goes on, the brain adapts to the use of ketone bodies for energy, and the scales are tipped in favour of a fat-derived energy source; up to 95% of energy production in starvation finally being derived from fat [10].

The net effect of this adaptation is to spare protein mass, and urinary nitrogen excretion falls from initial values of 8–10 g/24 hours to 2–4 g/24 hours over about two weeks [11].

As the period of starvation proceeds, the most important metabolic response of all occurs, namely a steady fall in basal energy requirements [12]. It is this adaptive process, when linked to the change in the source of energy, that is responsible for the prolonged survival seen in starvation.

It should not be forgotten that other metabolic problems occur in starvation. Mild acidosis [13] and hyperuricaemia are well documented [14]. Deficiencies of vitamins, haematinics and trace elements undoubtedly occur [15]. In the Belfast hunger strikers, neurological symptoms analogous to Wernicke's encephalopathy were reported [13].

Moreover, the above description applies to total starvation, and it is important in the context of nutritional support that this be appreciated, as the endocrine environment can change rapidly in response to refeeding [4]. Thus, if carbohydrate alone is administered (e.g. 5% dextrose infusions) insulin levels will rise, and its action will predominate. Thus lipolysis is inhibited and the use of ketones (ketosis) for energy will no longer be needed. Amino acid release from muscle will be inhibited [16] and the liver will be deprived of substrates for essential protein synthesis. Wernicke's encephalopathy or related neurological signs can be precipitated by administering 5% dextrose alone, either due to shortages of vitamins [17] or phosphate [18] required for glucose metabolism.

It follows, therefore, that a balanced nutritional formulation must be administered to starving patients, with great care being taken to replace depleted vitamin stores.

Injury

Classically, there are three phases of the metabolic response to injury (Table 5.3). The 'ebb' phase occurs immediately and is characterised primarily by an increase in catecholamine secretion [19]. The purpose of this part of the response is to allow escape to safety, and to maintain blood volume [4]. Glycogen is mobilised for immediate energy production and the metabolic rate falls [20]. This phase lasts no longer than 6–18 hours, even after severe injury. No thought need be given to nutritional

Table 5.3 Phases of the metabolic response to injury.

Phase	Duration	Role
Ebb	6–18 hours	Catecholamine secretion Maintenance of blood volume
Flow	5–60 days depending on type and severity of injury	Maintenance of energy production
Anabolic	Up to 30 days depending on type and severity of injury	Replacement of tissue lost in previous period

support during this period. The 'ebb' phase constitutes the immediate post-operative period following surgery, a time during which attention should be paid to achieving haemodynamic stability.

The 'flow' phase is the most important period where nutritional support is concerned. After uncomplicated elective surgery, it usually lasts five days or so, and is the time when the major metabolic changes providing energy occur. Weight loss is marked, and the energy requirements are increased. The whole philosophy of nutritional support in this phase should be to prevent as much tissue breakdown as possible by providing a balanced input of energy, nitrogen, trace elements and vitamins. It is important to emphasise that it is difficult to place patients in positive energy and nitrogen balance during this phase of the response, because of important compensatory hormonal changes that occur. In complicated injury, i.e. burns or surgery followed by protracted post-operative complications, the 'flow' phase may become prolonged, often for months.

In the third phase of the metabolic response to injury, the 'anabolic' phase, the so-called 'catabolic' hormonal response is reversed, and it becomes possible to place patients in overall positive energy and nitrogen balance. As the later text of this book will show, the expectations of nutritional support are often greater than seen in practice. This is usually because the clinician expects to place his patients in positive nitrogen balance in the 'flow' phase of the response to injury. Some knowledge of the metabolic responses that occur in the 'flow' phase should explain why nutritional support can only be expected to partially compensate for the breakdown of body tissue, rather than to rebuild it.

The 'flow' phase of injury (Table 5.4)

The most important aspect of the 'flow' phase of injury is that basal energy requirements increase and the basal metabolic rate rises, by as much as 25% after multiple fracture [21] and by 100% in severe burns [22]. This increased demand in energy is met, in part at least, by hormonal changes. Catecholamine secretion remains high for some time, dependent on the severity of the injury [23]. There is also excess production of glucagon [24], growth hormone [25] and cortisol [24]. Insulin secretion, initially inhibited in the 'ebb' phase by the high circulating catecholamine levels, returns, but there appears to be resistance to its actions [26], as both insulin and glucose levels are high.

These changes result in a mobilisation of adipose triglyceride and breakdown of muscle protein to provide energy from

Table 5.4 Metabolic changes in the 'flow' phase of the response to injury. Adapted from the data of [4].

Metabolic rate	Increased
Hormonal changes	Increases in
	Catecholamines
	Glucagon
	Cortisol
	Growth hormone
	Insulin*
Energy production	Protein and fat (maximum 80%)
Nitrogen	Losses increased
Water and sodium	Retention

* Insulin increased but with relative insulin deficiency on account of insulin resistance [26]

lipolysis, branched-chain amino acid oxidation in muscle and gluconeogenesis. In contrast to energy production in starvation, a maximum of only 80% of energy demands in the injured patient, can be derived from fat [27]. The remainder is met from protein breakdown. It follows from this discussion that weight loss in response to the increased energy demand in injury is marked, often up to 1.5 kg/24 hours. Recent work shows that this is not only caused by fat and protein breakdown, but also by diminished protein synthesis [28–31]. Moreover the increases in protein breakdown, as well as decreased protein synthesis, explain why nitrogen losses are so high in severe injury. It should not be forgotten that during muscle breakdown intracellular ions, including potassium, phosphorus and sulphur, are released to be excreted in the urine in fixed ratios to the amount of muscle protein catabolised [1].

EFFECTS OF NUTRITIONAL SUPPORT

At last a picture is emerging of the interactions between nutritional support, the degree of injury and nitrogen losses. Amino acid infusions in the post-operative period maintain the rate of protein synthesis [32], and detailed animal studies confirm the importance of an amino acid and energy supply to maintain or slightly increase protein synthesis rates in injury as compared with the control period [33]. Thus in the 'flow' phase of the metabolic response to severe injury, the gap between breakdown and synthesis can only be narrowed by providing nutritional support, mainly on account of increased synthesis rates. Overall positive nitrogen balance can only be achieved when the 'catabolic' hormonal response is reversed in the 'anabolic' phase of the response to injury, so that protein breakdown rates decrease and synthesis rates increase.

It might appear that the most beneficial results of nutritional support in the injured patient can be obtained in the 'anabolic' phase of the metabolic response as positive energy balance can usually be obtained fairly easily and the results may look good to the uninitiated observer. It is, however, a great deal more important to provide support to minimise net energy and nitrogen losses in the 'flow' phase, as this is the crucial period when the injured patient is hypermetabolic and losing large quantities of nitrogen and fat.

THE MIXED PICTURE OF INJURY AND STARVATION

As the metabolic changes in starvation are geared towards conserving energy output, whereas in response to injury the metabolic response is geared towards coping with the increased energy demands, it follows that the nutritional requirements of the starved and injured patient are markedly different.

In practice, many of the patients requiring nutritional support do not fall simply into one or other category. Frequently they may be injured after a period of under-nutrition (e.g. oesophagogastrectomy after a period of starvation due to mechanical dysphagia) or, unfortunately, prolonged under-nutrition following injury may occur (prolonged paralytic ileus following gastrointestinal surgery). It is as well to remember that the magnitude of the increased energy requirements in response to injury is governed largely by the size of the injury [34] but is markedly reduced at any given injury size by prior starvation [35, 36]. As will be discussed in more detail in Chapter 6, the magnitude of the metabolic response is usually best judged in the clinical setting by prospectively measuring urinary nitrogen losses. Since total nitrogen estimations are time consuming and relatively expensive, and the total urinary nitrogen loss is well reflected by that of urea [37], it is the urea excretion that is usually used. A correction may be made for changes in serum urea concentration [38], giving a better indication of the amount of urea produced.

Once estimates of nitrogen excretion have been made, an appropriate nutrition regime can be formulated based on these data (see Chapter 6).

REFERENCES

1   Cuthbertson D.P. (1930) The disturbance of metabolism produced by bony and non-bony injury, with notes on certain abnormal conditions of bone. *Biochem. J.* **24**, 1244.

2   Jones B.J.M., Lees R., Andrews J., Frost P. & Silk D.B.A. (1983) Comparison of an elemental and polymeric enteral diet in patients with normal gastrointestinal function. *Gut* **24**, 78.

3   Keohane P.P., Jones B.M.J. & Silk D.B.A. (1981) The roles of lactose and *C. difficile* in the pathogenesis of enteral feeding associated diarrhoea. *J. Parent. Ent. Nutr.* **5**, 359.

4   Woolfson A.M.J. (1979) Metabolic considerations in nutritional support. *Res. Clin. Forums* **1**, 35.

5   Cahill G.F. (1970) Starvation in man. *New Engl. J. Med.* **282**, 668.

6   Cahill G.F., Herrera M.G., Morgan A.P., *et al* (1968) Hormone-fuel interrelationships during fasting. *J. Clin. Invest.* **45**, 1751.

7   Levenson S.M., Barbul A. & Siefter E. (1977) Some biochemical, endocrinologic and immunologic changes and adaptations following starvation. In *Nutritional Aspects of Care in the Critically Ill*, eds. J.R. Richards and J.M. Kinney. Churchill Livingstone, Edinburgh.

8   Blackburn G.L. & Rienhoff H.Y. (1978) Isotonic crystalline amino acids for protein sparing. In *Advances in Parenteral Nutrition*, ed. I.D.A. Johnston, p. 119. MTP Press, Lancaster.

9   Felig P., Owen O.E, Wahren J. (1969) Amino acid metabolism during prolonged starvation. *J. Clin. Invest.* **48**, 584.

10 Grande F. (1968) Energetics and weight reduction. *Am. J. Clin. Nutr.* **21**, 305.

11 Benedict F.G. (1915) In *A Study of Prolonged Fasting*, Publication 203. Carnegie Institute, Washington DC.

12 Keys A., Brozek J., Henschel A., *et al* (1956) In *The Biology of Human Starvation*. University of Minnesota Press, Minneapolis.

13 Love A.H.G. (1982) Prolonged starvation. In *Extremes of Nutrition*. First British Society of Gastroenterology/Glaxo International Teaching Day.

14 Schatanoft J., Duncan T.G. & Duncan G.G. (1970) Effects of allopurinol on hyperuricaemia secondary to fasting. *Metabolism* **19**, 84.

15 Dickerson J.W.T. (1981) Vitamins and trace elements in the seriously ill patient. *Acta Chir. Scand.* Suppl 507, 144.

16 O'Connell R.C., Morgan A.P., Aoki T.T., *et al* (1974) Nitrogen conservation in starvation. Graded responses to intravenous glucose. *J. Clin. Endocrinol. Metabol.* **39**, 555.

17 Watson A.J.S., Walker J.F., Tomkin G.H., *et al* (1981) Acute Warnicke's encephalopathy precipitated by glucose loading. *Irish J. Med. Sci.* **150**, 301.

18 Silvis S.E., Di Bartolomeo A.G. & Aaker H.M. (1980) Hypophosphataemia and neurological changes secondary to oral calorie intake. *Am. J. Gastroenterol.* **73**, 215.

19 Coward R.F. & Smith P. (1966) Excretion of metanephrines in post-operative stress. *Clin. Chim. Acta* **14**, 832.

20 Stoner H.B. (1976) An integrated neuro-endocrine response to injury. In *Metabolism and the Response to Injury*, eds. A.W.

Wilkinson and D.P. Cuthbertson. Pitman Medical, Tunbridge Wells.

21 Cutherbertson D.P. (1982) Post shock metaloric response. *Lancet* **i**, 433.

22 Wilmore D.W., Long J.H., Mason A.D., *et al* (1974) Catecholamines: mediator of the hypermetabolic response to thermal injury. *Ann. Surg.* **180**, 653.

23 Birke G., Duner H., Liljedahl S.O., Pernow B., *et al* (1957) Histamine, catecholamines and adrenocortical steroids in burns. *Acta Chir. Scand.* **114**, 87.

24 Cope C., Nathanson I.T., Rourke G.M. & Wilson H. (1943) Metabolic observations on shock. *Ann. Surg.* **117**, 937.

25 Ross H., Johnston I.D.A., Welborn T.A. & Wright A.D. (1966) Effect of abdominal operation on glucose tolerance and serum levels of insulin, growth hormone and hydrocortisone. *Lancet* **ii**, 563.

26 Allison S.P., Hinton P. & Chamberlain M.J. (1968) Intravenous glucose tolerance, insulin and free fatty acid levels in burned patients. *Lancet* **ii**, 1113.

27 Kinney J.M., Duke J.M., Long C.L. & Gump F.E. (1970) Tissue fuel and weight loss after injury. *J. Clin. Pathol.* **23** (Suppl 4), 65.

28 Crane C.W., Picou D., Smith R. & Waterlow J.C. (1977) Protein turnover in patients before and after elective orthopaedic procedures. *Br. J. Surg.* **64**, 129.

29 Williamson D.H., Farrell R., Kerr A. & Smith R. (1977) Muscle-protein catabolism after injury in man, as measured by urinary excretion of 3-methyl histidine. *Clin. Sci.* **52**, 527.

30 O'Keefe S.J.D., Sender P.M. & James W.P.T. (1974) 'Catabolic' loss of body nitrogen in response to surgery. *Lancet* **ii**, 1035.

31 Bilmazes C., Kien C.L., Rohrbaugh D.K., *et al* (1978) Quantitative contribution of skeletal muscle to elevated rates of whole body protein breakdown in burned children as measured by N^{15}-methyl histidine output. *Metabolism* **27**, 671.

32 James W.P.T. (1981) Protein and energy metabolism after trauma. Old concepts and new developments. *Acta Chir. Scand.* Suppl 507, 1.

33 Stein T.P., Leskiw M.J., Wallace H.W. & Oram-Smith J.C. (1977) Changes in protein synthesis after trauma: importance of nutrition. *Am. J. Physics* **233**, E 348.

34 Moore F.D. (1959) In *Metabolic Care of the Surgical Patient.* W.B. Saunders, Philadelphia.

35 Abbott W.E. & Albertsen K. (1963) The effect of starvation, infection and injury on the metabolic processes and body composition. *Ann. NY Acad. Sci.* **110**, 941.

36 Munro H.N. & Cuthbertson D.P. (1943) The response of protein metabolism to injury. *Biochem. J.* **37**, 7.

37 Lee H.A. & Hartley T.F. (1975) A method of determining daily nitrogen requirements. *Postgrad. Med. J.* **51**, 441.

38 Peaston M.J.T. (1966) External metabolic balance studies during nasogastric feeding in serious illnesses requiring intensive care. *Br. Med. J.* **2**, 1367.

Chapter 6
Nutritional Requirements and Methods of Providing Nutritional Support

Once the decision has been reached that nutritional support is indicated, it remains to decide by which route nutrients should be administered. Table 6.1 summarises the variety of ways in which nutritional support can be provided. It is important to emphasise that gastrointestinal function is likely to be normal or near normal in most patients, so that the first option that has to be considered is whether nutrients can be administered directly to the gastrointestinal tract (enteral nutrition) or whether it will be necessary to resort to providing nutritional support via the intravenous route (parenteral nutrition).

There has been general agreement in the past that many patients have been managed unnecessarily via the parenteral route [1]. Although the two methods (enteral and parenteral nutrition) should be thought of as complementary, not competitive, parenteral nutrition should only be indicated when the enteral route is not viable [2].

As Chapter 7 will show, enteral nutrition can be provided in a number of ways, which include the administration of liquidised food, 'sip' feeding with palatable nutritional supplements, nasogastric and nasoenteric feeding, as well as administration of liquid diets via gastrostomies or feeding jejunostomies. In our experience, it is proving possible, with the aid of technological advances in administration methods, to feed an increasing proportion of patients via the enteral route. In the first formal

Table 6.1 Methods of providing nutritional support.

Enteral nutrition	Oral feeding
	Nasogastric feeding
	Nasoenteric feeding
	Gastrostomy
	Duodenostomy
	Jejunostomy
Parenteral nutrition	

retrospective analysis of our nutritional service, 76% of patients were fed exclusively via the enteral route.

Parenteral nutrition is approximately 10 times more expensive than enteral nutrition (£200–250 per week) and is associated with a higher incidence of serious side-effects. Nevertheless, as Table 6.2 shows, it has an important role to play in the management of severely ill patients [3].

OBJECTIVES AND EXPECTATIONS OF NUTRITIONAL SUPPORT

It should be appreciated from the outset that nutritional support is but one link in a chain of therapy for each patient. There is nothing magic about the effects of nutritional support on patient outcome, and the mortality in our series of parenteral and enteral nutrition is as high as 40% [4]. This point is still not completely understood, although we are now called far less frequently in the middle of the night to 'do' parenteral nutrition because a patient has become unexpectedly and acutely malnourished and the surgeons want to operate next day.

The overall aims of nutritional support should be to maintain organ function, promote healing, improve host defences against infection, strengthen the patient and thereby reduce morbidity and hasten mobility and convalescence [5].

The objectives will vary, however, according to the underlying metabolic status of each patient. Ideally, nutritional status should be maintained in the normally nourished patient and improved in

Table 6.2 Indications for total parenteral nutrition[1].

Definite benefit	Probable benefit
Management of short bowel syndrome[2]	Acute pancreatitis
Intestinal fistulas—without distal obstruction	Post-operatively—major surgery and complications
Intra-abdominal sepsis	
Major burns	*Benefit not proven*
Major sepsis	Adjunct to cancer
Adjunct to cancer	chemotherapy/radiotherapy
Multiple injuries involving viscera	Inflammatory bowel disease[3]
Pancreatic abscess/psuedocyst/ trauma/fistula	Pre-operatively—if weight loss > 10% of ideal weight

1 When enteral nutrition is inadequate or impossible
2 In conjunction with enteral nutrition to induce intestinal adaptation
3 Not as primary therapy

the nutritionally depleted patient. At the very least, the rate of reduction in protein and energy resources should be reduced to a minimum.

In practice, however, the achievement of the ideal objectives is limited by a number of factors (Table 6.3) and there will be differences between injury and starvation. Nutritionally depleted starving patients can be expected to show marked improvements in lean body mass and can even go into positive nitrogen balance when sufficient protein is given, despite low calorie intake; malnourished patients suffering the catabolic response to injury or sepsis may not show significant gains in lean body mass during nutritional therapy until the catabolic response ceases and the anabolic phase commences.

Table 6.3 lists the factors that together with poor feeding techniques and various specific nutritional deficiencies are associated with a delay in the onset of the anabolic phase and thus mitigate against the achievement of net protein synthesis.

During the catabolic phase, therefore, all that can be expected of nutritional support is the maintenance of lean body mass at its pre-therapy value, such that subsequent anabolism starts in the least malnourished state that is possible.

NUTRITIONAL REQUIREMENTS

Having decided to institute nutritional support, either by the enteral or parenteral route, the next step is to ensure that the nutritional requirements of each individual patient are met. As Table 6.4 shows, this means more than satisfying energy and nitrogen requirements, and includes meeting fluid, electrolyte, mineral, trace element and vitamin requirements. Although a lot of research has gone into formulating the composition of the commercially available enteric diets and parenteral nutrition solutions, deficiencies still occur commonly during treatment— for example 53% of 34 patients receiving nasogastrically administered Vivonex (Eaton Laboratories, Woking, Surrey) became hypokalaemic and 47% of the same group became hypophosphataemic during treatment [6].

Such deficiencies probably arise not only on account of inadequacies in diet formulation, but because established deficiencies precede treatment and/or because excessive losses occur on account of the underlying disease process. The exact nutritional requirements can therefore in reality only be determined by careful biochemical monitoring and subsequent supplementation of the nutritional regime.

Table 6.5 summarises the tentative nutritional requirements of patients requiring 8–20 g of nitrogen a day.

Table 6.3 Factors limiting achievements of nutritional objectives.

Most common	*Common*
Sepsis	Technique
Trauma	Insufficient energy supply
Severe fractures	Insufficient amino-nitrogen supply
Major visceral injury	Insufficient cofactors for nitrogen utilisation
Major burns	Fluid balance
Major operations	Inability to tolerate volume required for
Immobility	nutritional requirements
Bedbound	
Splintage of fractures	*Unusual*
Neurological causes	Metabolic
Muscle relaxant drugs in intensive care	Hyperglycaemia unresponsive to insulin
Pain	Hyponatraemia due to inappropriate
	antidiuretic hormone secretion
	Occult losses of protein
	Low ambient temperature

Energy

Nitrogen

Fluid

Electrolytes

Minerals

Trace elements

Vitamins—water and fat soluble

Table 6.5   A guide to the daily nutritional requirements for enteral and parenteral nutrition.

	Nitrogen	8–20 g
	Energy	1500–4000 kcal
Electrolytes	Sodium	70–150 mmol
	Chloride	70–220 mmol
	Potassium	50–100 mmol
	Calcium	5–10 mmol
	Magnesium	5–20 mmol
	Phosphate	40–50 mmol

Energy and nitrogen

There is a close relationship between energy and nitrogen balance, such that the two must always be considered jointly [7].

Unless non-protein energy equal to total metabolic expenditure is supplied, weight loss will occur. Energy is therefore required to provide for the patient's basal metabolic rate plus suprabasal requirements that include:

1   Activity.

2   Nutrient intake (specific dynamic action).

3   Environmental temperature.

Resting metabolism can be measured clinically by indirect calorimetry. Assessments can also be made, either by use of nomograms using height and weight or by Kleiber's formula [8]:

$$\text{Energy requirements (kcal/day)} = 70 \times (\text{body weight kg})^{\frac{3}{4}}$$

A useful working figure of 25 kcal/kg per day satisfies the basal requirements for normal adults, and for most adult patients receiving nutritional support energy requirements can be satisfied by an intake of 40–50 kcal/kg per day, equivalent to 3000 kcal or so for a 70 kg patient. As Table 6.6 shows, several factors affect energy expenditure, and must be accounted for when formulating nutritional regimes. It is as well to appreciate that most operative procedures do not result in an increased energy expenditure of more than 10% [9]. However, certain conditions such as multiple fractures, severe sepsis or peritonitis and large area burns, are associated with greater increases in resting energy expenditure of 30–100% or more.

The relationship between nitrogen and energy intake and nitrogen balance is such that for a given energy intake increasing nitrogen intake results in an improvement in nitrogen balance up to a certain point, above which no further effect is seen.

The relationship holds for whatever energy intake is supplied, but overall positive nitrogen balance can only be achieved if energy intake is in excess of total requirements. Although data from studies in normal active men shows that positive nitrogen balance could be attained, even with an energy intake below metabolic requirements [10], investigations carried out in patients receiving nutritional support highlight the benefits in respect of achieving positive nitrogen balance with provisions of energy in excess of metabolic requirements [11–13].

Although the absolute requirement of energy for optional utilisation of ingested nitrogen holds true in all clinical circum-

Table 6.6 Factors affecting energy expenditure.

	Change in energy expenditure
Starvation	−
Sepsis	+
Physical activity	+
Paralysis	−
Core temperature rise	+13% per °C
Heat losses	
Low ambient temperature	+
Burns	+
Low humidity	+
Diminished body mass	−
Injury	
Elective uncomplicated surgery	+10%
Major elective surgery	+15–20%
Multiple fractures	+10–20%
Septicaemia/peritonitis	+20–50%
Large area burns	+30–125%

+ increases
− decreases

stances, the relative requirements of each (i.e. the ratio of non-protein energy to nitrogen or 'calorie to nitrogen' ratio) varies. Thus, as Table 6.7 shows, positive nitrogen balance in active man can be achieved at a nitrogen intake of 8–9 g/24 hour with an energy intake of approximately 3000 non-protein kcals, giving a non-protein to nitrogen ratio of 325 kcal/g N.

Starved patients have a greater capacity of nitrogen retention than normals [14], and positive nitrogen balance can be attained with a nitrogen intake as low as 7 g and a non-protein energy intake of some 1800 kcal with a ratio of 250 kcal/g.

There is much less certainty, however, about the requirements of patients receiving nutritional support with marked and modest increases in energy expenditure. The requirements shown in Table 6.7 are those assessed by Woolfson [7]. In patients with modest increases in energy expenditure, requirements of 14 g nitrogen and 3000 kcal non-protein energy intake with a ratio of approximately 200 kcal/g nitrogen are quoted. The latest work from Hill's group in Leeds suggests that in parenterally fed surgical patients, nitrogen equilibrium (i.e. no net gain or loss) can be achieved with such an intake of nitrogen (0.3 g N/kg per day) but with a ratio of 150 kcal/g nitrogen [15]. To achieve significant positive nitrogen balance, however, their inference is that both nitrogen and energy intake has to be increased [16] over and above the figures quoted by Woolfson [7], although it is possible that future studies will indicate that net gains in protein synthesis can be achieved in such patients with rather more modest increases in energy expenditure by maintaining a high intake of nitrogen, but accompanied with a lower ratio of energy to nitrogen in the region of 135 kcal/g N, the figure usually quoted for the hypermetabolic group of patients [16].

In patients with very high resting energy expenditure, there is general agreement that they have high nitrogen requirements, often up to 22–25 g nitrogen per day. Relatively speaking, they

Table 6.7 Approximate requirements for energy and nitrogen in different patients. Based on data in [7].

| | Basal metabolic requirements | | |
	Normal	Moderate increase	Markedly raised
Nitrogen (g/24 hours)	7.5	14	25
Energy (kcal/24 hours)	2000	3000	4000
Non-protein energy: nitrogen ratio (kcal/g)	250	200	135

have lower energy requirements, with ratios as low as 125 kcal/g nitrogen [14, 17, 18]. It needs to be re-emphasised, though, that it is often difficult to achieve positive nitrogen balance in patients with very high resting expenditure, and the best that can often be expected of nutritional support in these patients is the maintenance of protein stores at pre-therapy values, such that when energy requirements fall and it becomes possible to achieve positive nitrogen balance, the patient is in the least malnourished state that is possible [3].

Carbohydrate or fat as the energy source?

The nature of the non-protein energy source that should be employed in nutritional support remains the subject of continuing debate and controversy. Most of the studies performed to date have concerned patients receiving parenteral rather than enteral nutrition, so the conclusions drawn are not necessarily applicable to the area of enteral nutrition.

In the severely ill patient with high energy expenditure and nitrogen requirements in excess of 18 g nitrogen per day, evidence has been presented suggesting that there is a lack of stimulation of endogenous lipid metabolism [12, 19, 20] caused, it is thought, by associated hormonal changes with resultant low levels of free fatty acids and ketones and high levels of glucose, lactate and insulin [20]. Insulin, it will be remembered, exerts an anti-lipolytic effect [7]. In these circumstances, the use of fat emulsions as the energy source would not be expected to exert their expected nitrogen sparing effect and, there are now clinical studies to show that the limited nitrogen sparing effect of fat emulsions in such patients is related to utilisation of the glycerol and not the fatty acid content of the fat emulsions used [21].

Other patients with high energy expenditures in whom, despite their ability to mobilise fat stores in response to stress, anaerobic metabolism may predominate [19], concomitantly produce lactate and convert acetyl-CoA to ketone bodies (acetoacetate, β-hydroxybutyrate and acetone) rather than allow entry into the tricarboxylic acid cycle. High blood ketones stimulate insulin secretion [7], with concomitant inhibition of lipolysis [22]. This is the stage at which the patient is said to be fully 'keto-adapted', and this being the case one could certainly infer that any extra fat administered could not be handled.

In the light of these observations, we recommend that patients requiring more than 18–20 g nitrogen per day should receive a carbohydrate-based, rather than lipid-based, energy source. Again, these recommendations would apply mainly to patients on parenteral rather than enteral nutrition, as equivalent data is not available for the latter patients. To avoid the onset of essential fatty acid deficiency, all patients should receive the equivalent of 4% of total calories as triglyceride, although this can be quite safely administered once a week.

In patients with more modest energy expenditure and nitrogen requirements, the latest studies indicate that better protein repletion is obtained if an energy source based upon fat and carbohydrate is used [15]. Although a number of previous studies had suggested that when glucose is used as an energy source nitrogen is retained just as well [12, 23, 24], if not better [21, 25, 26], than with equicaloric amounts of fat administered together with glucose, the data from Leeds [15] were obtained from patients who received parenteral nutrition for longer periods than in the studies where glucose alone was associated with better nitrogen retention [21, 25, 26]. We therefore routinely use an energy source based upon fat and carbohydrate in our patients requiring nutritional support who have modest energy expenditures and nitrogen requirements of less than 18 g/day.

CALCULATING THE ENERGY AND NITROGEN REQUIREMENTS

As mentioned on p. 55, the energy and nitrogen requirements can be calculated from the energy requirements. Basal energy requirements are calculated first from the formula, and appropriate corrections made for increases in requirements that occur in response to injury (Table 6.6). Nitrogen requirements can then be matched according to the standard values in Table 6.7.

Alternatively, and more simply, nitrogen losses can be assessed in the urine, faeces, fistula or drain fluids, or may be calculated from measurement of urine urea excretion, thus:

$$\text{Nitrogen loss} = \text{mmol urinary urea (g/24 hours)}/24 \text{ hours} \times 0.028 + 2$$

+2 represents an approximation of non-urinary urea losses. Requirements may be calculated to exceed losses by 3–5 g nitrogen/day in non-catabolic patients and to match losses in catabolic patients, with the non-protein energy requirements estimated from Table 6.7.

WATER AND ELECTROLYTES

The fluid and electrolyte requirements have to be assessed on an individual patient basis and the values quoted in Table 6.5 act as guidelines only. As a general principle, biological fluids should be collected daily from appropriate orifices of sick patients (e.g.

gastric aspirates, fistula and drain effluents, urine, diarrhoeal faeces) and analysed for fluid and electrolyte content and appropriate supplementations made. Insensible losses should be estimated and taken into account [27].

Sodium

The content of sodium in the different nutritional preparations is variable and note should be taken of this when calculating requirements. Diets or parenteral solutions high in sodium are useful in situations of increased sodium need, such as high fistula losses. Specially formulated diets and solutions with low sodium content are now available for patients in need of sodium restriction, such as in renal failure or advanced parenchymal liver disease (see Chapters 9, 10).

Potassium

Hypokalaemia is the most common deficiency that arises in our patients receiving nutritional support and develops in 50% of patients at some stage during therapy. Analysis of tissue indicates that approximately 3 mmol K^+ is present for each gram of nitrogen. K^+ is the major intracellular ion, and during catabolism losses occur in a fixed ratio to nitrogen. Similarly in the anabolic phase, during synthesis of muscle mass, K^+ moves from the intravascular space into the intracellular pool so that hypokalaemia develops if insufficient K^+ is administered with nitrogen. At least 5 mmol K^+ should probably be administered with each gram of nitrogen [28].

Phosphate

If inadequate phosphate is given, particularly when glucose is used as an energy source, profound hypophosphataemia may occur [29]. Hypophosphataemia causes falls in levels of ATP and of 2,3-diphosphoglycerate [30], and in severe deficiency states neurological symptoms, including dysarthria, parasthesiae, disorentiation fitting and coma, can occur [3]. It is usually stated that the daily phosphate requirements are in the region of 30 mmol [5, 7]. We think this may be an under-estimation and usually administer 40–60 mmol.

OTHER ELECTROLYTE AND TRACE ELEMENTS

Although normal daily requirements of many of the electrolytes and trace elements have been established, it must be appreciated that many patients requiring nutritional support may have become deficient, prior to treatment, not only due to previous under-nutrition, but also on account of the nature of the underlying illness, e.g. prolonged diarrhoea [31]. The daily calcium requirements are in the region of 5–10 mmol/day and levels should be monitored at least weekly, as long-term nutritional support has led to overt rickets and osteomalacia. Magnesium deficiency may induce muscular fibrillation and should be suspected in patients with prolonged diarrhoea (e.g. Crohn's disease).

The human body contains approximately 40 elements. Of these the 'major' elements constitute 99% of the body composition (H, Na, Mg, K, Ca, C, N, O, P, S, Cl). Those remaining are present in such minute amounts that, until recently, they could not be determined accurately and were described as trace elements. At least nine trace elements (Table 6.8), and possibly five others (nickel, tin, vanadium, silicone and fluoride), are considered essential for optimum health [32].

Iron, iodine and cobalt are the trace elements which have received most attention historically. Their metabolism is reasonably well understood and they have established themselves in clinical therapeutics. Iodine and cobalt function solely as components of the thyroid hormones and vitamin B12 respectively, and failure of intake leads to specific abnormalities. Although iron is involved in cytochrome respiration, it is overwhelmingly

Table 6.8 Trace elements considered to be essential.

Element	Deficiency syndrome	Estimated daily requirements
Iron	Anaemia	10–18 mg [32]
Iodine	Hypothyroidism	10–200 μg [32]
Cobalt	Vitamin B12 deficiency	1.5–40 mg [32]
Zinc	Eczematous dermatitis, lethargy, anaemia, diarrhoea [33]	3–15 mg [35]
Selenium	Cardiomyopathy [39]	100–200 μg [3]
Copper	Anaemia, leukopenia, neutropenia, skeletal abnormalities [40, 41]	0.3–0.5 mg [42]
Chromium	Impaired glucose tolerance, neuropathy [43]	50–200 μg [32]
Molybdenum	Amino acid intolerance [44]	150–500 μg [32]
Managanese	—	2–3 mg [45]
Vanadium	Salt and water retention [33]	—

required for haemoglobin synthesis. Deficiencies of these elements are easily and specifically recognised because the vulnerable pool of each is known, large and accessible. For none of the other elements do we know, with any certainty, the vulnerable metabolically active fraction [33]. We thus know less about requirements, and the specific clinical deficiency syndromes have not been fully characterised. In this regard, however, long-term nutritional support, particularly parenteral nutrition, has produced a crop of reports of deficiencies.

Zinc deficiency has often been described in patients receiving nutritional support [34]. Clinically patients present with an eczematous dermatitis, similar to that seen in acrodermatitis enteropathica, a rare congenital defect of zinc absorption. Affected patients also often appear lethargic and develop diarrhoea and anaemia. Recent studies in patients receiving parenteral nutrition have emphasised the importance of zinc metabolism in relationship to nitrogen balance [35]. There does not seem to be a functional body store of zinc; virtually all the zinc is locked in bone or protein, which explains not only the rapidity of onset of symptoms on a zinc-deficient diet but also the rapidity of response to dietary supplementation. Although it follows that measurement of the plasma zinc level does not accurately reflect tissue levels, plasma measurements still provide the only convenient method of assessment, and if plasma levels are low supplements should be given. Finally, it should be mentioned that zinc deficiency *per se* may lead to poor wound healing [36], and an increased susceptibility to infections, mediated in part, it is thought, by defects in cellular mediated immunity [37].

Selenium is a component of glutathione peroxidase [38], an enzyme which reduces toxic lipid peroxides to hydroxy-acids. In the absence of selenium lipid peroxides and free radicles may damage cell membranes. A patient on a long-term selenium-deficient parenteral nutrition regime has been reported to have died of a cardiomyopathy [39], the histology of which closely resembled the myocardial damage in animals on selenium-deficient diets and in humans with selenium-deficient cardiomyopathy in China (Keshan's disease).

Copper plays an important role in iron absorption and transport, is essential for normal development of the skeleton, for normal function and structure of the central nervous system, for taste sensation and for pigmentation [40]. Copper deficiency in patients receiving parenteral nutrition has been associated with anaemia (microcytic, hypochromic), leucopenia, neutropenia and skeletal abnormalities [41]. The copper requirements in parenteral nutrition have now been defined [42].

Impaired glucose intolerance and neuropathy have been

described in a patient on long-term parenteral nutrition, both of which were reversed by chromium infusion [43].

Molybdenum deficiency may be associated with amino acid intolerance [44]. Little is known about the clinical syndrome of manganese deficiency.

Although estimates of daily requirements have been given in Table 6.8, the absolute requirements during nutritional support are not known with any certainty. For patients on short-term nutritional support, occasional supplements should be given, more to replete potential deficiencies that might have arisen on account of the underlying disease state. Regular supplements should, however, be administered to *all* patients receiving nutritional support for longer than a month.

VITAMIN REQUIREMENTS (Table 6.9)

Requirements will depend on the clinical state of the patient and will vary according to the degree of deficiency state prior to feeding and the type of injury sustained by the patient. Vitamins, as well as trace elements, make important contributions to metabolic processes, and it is likely that the requirements of all seriously ill patients are, as a whole, higher than those of healthy individuals. Requirements cannot be measured, so vitamin supplementation is necessary during enteral and parenteral nutrition, particularly when treatment is prolonged.

Table 6.9 Vitamin requirements. Modified from *Drug. Ther. Bull.* [52].

	Vitamin	Recommended daily intake (mg)
Water soluble	Thiamine (B1)	1.4
	Riboflavin (B2)	2.1
	Pyridoxine (B6)	2.1
	Cyanocobalamine (B12)	2.0
	Nicotinamide	14
	Biotin	0.4
	Pantothenic acid/ dexpanthenol	14
	Folic acid	2
	Ascorbic acid (C)	35
Fat soluble	Calciferol (D)	100 IU
	Phytylmenaquinone (K)	140 μg
	Retinol (A)	700 IU
	Tocopheryl acetate (E)	30 IU

Ascorbic acid may play a specific role in wound healing [46]. Surgery leads to an increased demand for ascorbic acid [47], and supplements should be given prior to surgery, as the interchange between plasma and tissues is slow [48].

Thiamine deficiency appears now to be common in elderly patients [46], particularly those undergoing surgery [49]. Alcoholics may be thiamine deficient; carbohydrate infusions may unmask thiamine deficiency in these patients. Supplements are therefore required to prevent development of the Wernicke–Korsakoff syndrome [3].

Folate depletion may occur quite commonly during parenteral nutrition [31], and may lead to acute pancytopenia, jaundice and impaired protein synthesis by interference with methionine metabolism [50].

Although supplements of the fat soluble vitamins A, D, E and K should be given, the positions of vitamins A and D are currently the subject of review. Excessive vitamin A and D administration in short-term treatment may give rise to exfoliative dermatitis and hypercalcaemia respectively [31]. Long-term parenteral nutrition has led to overt rickets and osteomalacia. However, a further syndrome associated with long-term parenteral nutrition includes hypercalcaemia, hypercalcuria and low parathyroid hormone levels in conjunction with a clinical and histological picture of osteomalacia. This paradoxically responds to a withdrawal of vitamin D [51].

REFERENCES

1   Bethal R.A., Jansen R.D., Heymsfield S.B., *et al* (1979) Nasogastric hyperalimentation through a polyethylene catheter. An alternative to central venous hyperalimentation. *Am. J. Clin. Nutr.* **32**, 1112.

2   Lee H.A. (1979) Why enteral nutrition? *Res. Clin. Forums* **1**, 15.

3   Jones B.J.M. & Silk D.B.A. (1982) Parenteral nutrition. *Med. Int.* **1**, 674.

4   Keohane P.P., Attrill H., Jones B.J.M., *et al* (1983) Influence of lactose and *C. difficile* on enteral feeding associated diarrhoea. *Clin Nutr.* (in press).

5   Powell-Tuck J. & Goode A.W. (1981) Principles of enteral and parenteral nutrition. *Br. J. Anaesthesia* **53**, 169.

6   Jones B.J.M., Lees R., Andrews J., Frost P. & Silk D.B.A. (1983) Comparison of an elemental and polymeric diet in patients with normal gastrointestinal function. *Gut* **24**, 78.

7   Woolfson A.M.J. (1979) Metabolic considerations in nutritional support. *Res. Clin. Forums* **1**, 33.

8   Wilmore D.W. (1977) *The Metabolic Management of the Critically Ill.* Plenum Medical, New York.

9   Kinney J.M., Duke J.H., Long C.L. & Gump F.E. (1970) Tissue fuel and weight loss after injury. *J. Clin. Pathol.* **23** (Suppl. 65).

10   Calloway D.H. & Spector H. (1954) Nitrogen balance as related to calorie and protein intake in active young men. *Am. J. Clin. Nutr.* **2**, 405.

11   Fitzpatric G.F., Meguid M.M., O'Connell R.C., *et al* (1975) Nitrogen sparing by carbohydrate in man: intermittent and continuous enteral compared with parenteral glucose. *Surgery* **78**, 105.

12   Jeejeebhoy K.N., Anderson G.H., Nakhooda A.F., *et al* (1976) Metabolic studies in total parenteral nutrition with lipid in man. *J. Clin. Invest.* **57**, 125.

13   Long J.M., Wilmore D.W., Mason A.D. & Pruitt B.A. (1974) Fat carbohydrate interaction. Nitrogen sparing effect of various caloric sources for total intravenous feeding. *Surg. Forum.* **25**, 61.

14   Wilmore D.W. (1977) *Energy requirements for maximum nitrogen retention.* Presented at the AMA Symposium, Amino Acid Metabolism, Denver, Colorado.

15   Macfie J., Smith R.C. & Hill G.L. (1981) Glucose or fat as a non-protein energy source. *Gastroenterology* **80**, 103.

16   Smith R.C., Burkinsaw L. & Hill G.L. (1982) Optimal energy and nitrogen intake for gastroenterological patients requiring intravenous nutrition. *Gastroenterology* **82**, 145.

17   Moore F.D. (1959) In *Metabolic Care of the Surgical Patient.* W.B. Saunders, Philadelphia.

18   Soroff H.S., Pearson E. & Artz C.P. (1961) An estimation of the nitrogen requirements for equilibrium in burned patients. *Surg. Gynaec. Obstet.* **112**, 159.

19   Holliday R.L., Viidik T. & Jennings B. (1978) Lipid metabolism in stress. In *Advances in Parenteral Nutrition*, ed. I.D.A. Johnston, p. 179. MTP Press, Lancaster.

20   O'Donnell T.F., Clowes G.H., Blackburn G.L., *et al* (1976) Proteolysis associated with a deficit of peripheral energy fuel substrates in septic man. *Surgery* **80**, 191.

21   Long J.M., Wilmore D.W., Mason A.D. & Pruitt B.A. (1977) Effect of carbohydrate and fat intake on nitrogen excretion during intravenous feeding. *Ann. Surg.* **185**, 417.

22   Blackburn G.L., Flatt J.P. & Hensle T.W. (1976) Peripheral amino acid infusions. In *Total Parenteral Nutrtion*, ed. J.E. Fischer, p. 363. Little Brown, Boston.

23   Bark S., Holm I., Hakarsson I. & Wretlind A. (1976) Nitrogen sparing effect of fat emulsion compared with glucose in postoperative period. *Acta Chir. Scand.* **142**, 423.

24   Gazzaniga A.B., Bartlett R.H. & Shobe J.B. (1975) Nitrogen balance in patients receiving either fat or carbohydrate for total intravenous nutrition. *Ann. Surg.* **182**, 163.

25   Woolfson A.M.J., Healey R.V. & Allison S.P. (1979) Insulin to inhibit protein catabolism after injury. *New Engl. J. Med.* **300**, 14.

26   Brennan M.F., Fitzpatrick G.F., Cohen K.H. & Moore F.D. (1975) Glycerol: major contributor to the short term protein sparing effect of fat emulsions in normal man. *Ann. Surg.* **182**, 386.

27   Peaston M.J.T. (1967) The maintenance of metabolism during intensive patient care. *Postgrad. Med. J.* **43**, 317.

28   Frost P.M. & Smith J.C. (1953) Influence of potassium salts on efficiency of parenteral protein alimentation in the surgical patient. *Metabolism* **2**, 529.

29 Groen J., Willebrands A.F., Kamminga C.E., *et al* (1952) Effects of glucose administration on the potassium and inorganic phosphate content of the blood serum and the electrocardiogram in normal individuals and in non-diabetic patients. *Acta Med. Scand.* **141**, 352.

30 Travis S.F., Sugerman H.J., Ruberg A.L., *et al* (1971) Alterations of red-cell glycolytic intermediates and oxygen transport as a consequence of hypophosphataemia in patients receiving intravenous hyperalimentation. *New Engl. J. Med.* **285**, 763.

31 Anonymous (1978) Deficiencies in parenteral nutrition. *Br. Med. J.* **2**, 913.

32 Aggett P.J. (1979) Trace elements in medicine. *Hosp. Update* **5**, 981.

33 Golden M.H.N. & Golden B.E. (1981) Trace elements. Potential importance in human nutrition with particular reference to zinc and vanadium. *Br. Med. Bull.* **37**, 31.

34 Kay R.G. & Tasman-Jones C. (1975) Zinc deficiency and intravenous feeding. *Lancet* **ii**, 605.

35 Wolman S.L., Anderson G.H., Marliss E.B., *et al* (1979) Zinc in total parenteral nutrition: requirements and metabolic effects. *Gastroenterology* **76**, 458.

36 Golden M.H.N., Golden B.E. & Jackson A.A. (1978) Skin breakdown in kwashiorkor response to zinc. *Lancet* **i**, 1256.

37 Golden M.H.N., Golden B.E., Harland P.S.E.G. & Jackson A.A. (1978) Zinc and immunocompetence in protein-energy malnutrition. *Lancet* **i**, 1226.

38 Ganther H.E., Hafeman D.G., Lawrence R.A., *et al* (1976) In *Trace Elements in Human Health and Disease*, Vol. 2, ed. A.S. Prasad, p. 165. Academic Press, New York.

39 Fleming C.R., Lie J.T., McCall J.T., *et al* (1982) Selenium deficiency and fatal cardiomyopathy in a patient on home parenteral nutrition. *Gastroenterology* **83**, 689.

40 Ashkenazi A., Levin S., Djaldetti M. *et al* (1973) The syndrome of neonatal copper deficiency. *Pediatrics* **52**, 525.

41 Vilter R.W., Bozian R.C. & Hess E.V. (1974) Manifestations of copper deficiency in a patient with systemic sclerosis on intravenous hyperalimentation. *New Engl. J. Med.* **291**, 188.

42 Shike M., Roulet M., Kurian R., *et al* (1981) Copper metabolism and requirements in total parenteral nutrition. *Gastroenterology* **81**, 290.

43 Jeejeebhoy K.M., Chu R., Marliss E.B., *et al* (1975) Chromium deficiency, diabetes and neuropathy, reversed by chromium infusion in a patient on total parenteral nutrition (TPN) for $3\frac{1}{2}$ years. *Clin. Res.* **23**, 636A.

44 Abumrad N.N. (1981) Amino acid intolerance during prolonged total parenteral nutrition reversed by molybdenum. *Clin. Res.* **27**, 621A.

45 Fell G.S. & Burns R.R. (1978) Zinc and other trace elements. In *Advances in Parenteral Nutrition*, ed. I.D.A. Johnston, p. 241. MTP Press, Lancaster.

46 Dickerson J.W.T. (1981) Vitamins and trace elements in the seriously ill patient. *Acta Chir. Scand.* Suppl 507, 144.

47 Crandon J.H., Lennihan R. Jr, Mikal S. & Reif A.E. (1961) Ascorbic acid economy in surgical patients. *Ann. NY Acad. Sci.* **92**, 246.

48   Katakity M. (1978) Some effects of nutritional supplement in elderly patients. MPhil Thesis, University of Surrey.

49   Older M.W.J., Edwards D. & Dickerson J.W.T. (1980) Studies of the effects of surgery on nutritional status with particular reference to vitamin status. Unpublished observations.

50   Connor H., Newton D.J., Preston F.E. & Woods H.F. (1978) Oral methionine loading as a cause of acute folate deficiency: its relevance to parenteral nutrition. *Postgrad. Med. J.* **54**, 318.

51   Allam B.F., Dryburgh F.J. & Sheakin A. (1981) Metabolic base disease during parenteral nutrition. *Lancet* **i**, 385.

52   Anonymous (1980) Adult parenteral nutrition: which preparations? *Drug Ther. Bull.* **18**, 85.

Chapter 7
Enteral Feeding

It is important to re-emphasise the fact that most patients requiring nutritional support have normal or near normal gastrointestinal function. Consequently, in all these patients attempts should be made to administer nutrients via the enteral rather than parenteral route. Apart from the cost factors involved (parenteral feeding is approximately ten times more expensive than enteral feeding), the complications that can develop during parenteral nutrition are more serious than those associated with enteral nutrition.

In the overall context of nutritional support, enteral nutrition can be defined as the administration of nutrients to patients via the gastrointestinal tract and, as Table 7.1 shows, there are, broadly speaking, three ways in which this can be achieved. First, liquidised food can be given orally to patients not able to ingest solid food. Examples of suitable patients are those who have problems with mastication and those with mechanical dysphagia to solid foods.

Secondly, palatable enteric diets can be administered orally as nutritional supplements to patients who are eating insufficient quantities of normal food. Suitable patients are usually those in whom anorexia is a prominent feature of the underlying illness. Finally, a wide range of enteric diets can be administered to patients via feeding tubes placed in the stomach, duodenum or small bowel. We have found this to be the most effective way of providing nutritional support via the enteral route, and most of our patients receiving enteral nutrition are fed in this way.

Once the decision is made to provide nutritional support via the enteral route, the best formulation to meet the nutritional needs of the individual patient must be selected. Although there are now a number of commercially available enteric diets, important differences exist in respect of their nutritional components. Knowledge gained about the processes involved in the normal physiology of nutrient absorption has formed the basis of the formulation of many of the preparations recommended for use in patients with normal gastrointestinal function. In contrast, a good deal of speculation has gone into formulating some of the preparations that are claimed to be of benefit to those patients with impaired gastrointestinal function. A brief insight into the physiological processes involved in nutrient absorption is therefore helpful, not only in understanding the rationale underlying diet formulation, but also in choosing the correct type of diet to satisfy individual nutritional requirements.

THE PHYSIOLOGY OF NUTRIENT ABSORPTION

Table 7.2 shows that the site of absorption of different nutrients varies. Thus while fat, carbohydrate, protein, iron and folic acid, as well as the bulk of water and electrolytes, are absorbed in the upper small intestine [1], vitamin B12, bile acids, and some water and electrolytes are absorbed in the ileum. Of relevance to enteral nutrition is the fact that the mechanisms for absorption of carbohydrate, protein, water and electrolytes are present in the

Table 7.1 Methods of providing nutritional support.

Route	Nutritional source
Oral feeding	Food Liquidised food Palatable enteral diet
Tube feeding Nasogastric Nasoduodenal Nasojejunal	Enteral diets Enteral diet
Gastrostomy	Liquidised food Enteral diet
Jejunostomy	Enteral diet

Table 7.2 Sites of nutrient absorption.

Nutrient	Site of absorption
Fat	Jejunum
Carbohydrate	Jejunum
Protein	Jejunum
Water and electrolytes	Jejunum (ileum, colon)
Iron	Duodenum
Folic acid	Jejunum
Vitamin B12	Ileum
Bile acids	Ileum

ileum as well as the jejunum, so that if the proximal jejunum is resected or diseased, normal absorption of these nutrients can still occur. Although it is usually stated that fat is absorbed in the jejunum [1], absorption of large quantities of fat probably takes place in the ileum as well, since steatorrhoea may occur when more than 100 cm of ileum are resected [2]. Therefore, in certain clinical situations where significant lengths of small intestine have been resected, enteric diets containing only small amounts of triglyceride may be indicated to prevent steatorrhoea from occurring. The absorption of folic acid and iron is probably restricted to the upper small intestine, so supplementation with these two haematinics will be required if the absorptive capacity of this region of the intestine is reduced. Similarly, vitamin B12 is absorbed only in the distal ileum, and in the absence of this region of the small intestine vitamin B12 supplementation will be required.

Fat absorption

Triglycerides, cholesterol and the fat-soluble vitamins A, D, E and K constitute the major dietary lipids. Daily adult intake of triglycerides varies (60–80 g) as does cholesterol (0.5–1 g). Triglycerides are triesters of glycerol (Fig. 5.1). Most contain fatty acids with 16–18 carbon atoms (long chain triglycerides), and are insoluble in water. Some contain fatty acids with 8–12 carbon atoms (medium chain triglycerides, MCT) and are more soluble. The process of absorption of dietary lipid is complicated and involves a number of steps, as described below.

1   *Intraluminal phase.* Dietary lipid is emulsified in the stomach by mechanical means and a coarse emulsion passes into the duodenum, where mixing with bile and pancreatic juice occurs. Glycerolesterhydrolase, commonly called lipase, is secreted by the pancreas. This enzyme hydrolyses the 1- and 3-esterbonds of the triglyceride molecule (Fig. 7.1), thereby producing free fatty acids and a 2-monoglyceride. Further hydrolysis of the 2-monoglyceride occurs, but only after isomerisation of the fatty acid to the 1 position has taken place. Cholesterol esters are hydrolysed by pancreatic cholesterol esterase.

2   *Micellar solubilisation.* The products of luminal lipid hydrolysis—free cholesterol, monoglycerides and fatty acids—are poorly soluble in the water milieu of the gut lumen and, as such, diffuse very slowly across the unstirred water layer, the limiting barrier between the bulk water phase of the lumen and the surface of mucosal cells. Efficient absorption requires that these products be

solubilised to allow more rapid movement to absorptive sites. Solubilisation is mediated by bile acids, the end-products of hepatic cholesterol metabolism. These are secreted in bile as peptide conjugates of glycine and taurine; as such they are readily soluble in jejunal contents (pH 6–7), since at this pH they are heavily ionised. Above a certain concentration, known as the critical micellar concentration (CMC), bile salts form molecular aggregates, known as pure bile salt micelles. Each molecule is orientated in such a way that the hydrophilic polar hydroxyl and amino groups face outwards and the non polar ends face inwards. The lipid soluble fatty acids, monoglycerides and phospholipids (derivatives of glycerol present in bile and the diet) are incorpor-

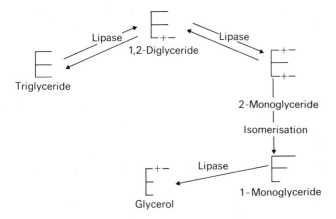

Fig. 7.1 Intraluminal hydrolysis of triglycerides by pancreatic lipase.

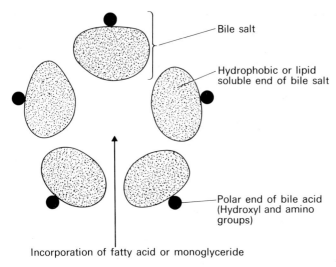

Incorporation of fatty acid or monoglyceride

Fig. 7.2 Schematic representation of the micelle.

ated into the hydrophobic core of the aggregate to form mixed micelles (Fig. 7.2). Due to the fact that these molecular aggregates have an outer rim of polar water soluble hydroxyl and amino groups, they are able to diffuse easily across the unstirred water layer. In this way the products of lipolysis packaged in the core of the micelle reach the surface of the intestinal microvilli, and by virtue of their lipid solubility are able to traverse the lipid membrane and enter the mucosal cells. Cholesterol and the fat soluble vitamins are readily incorporated into mixed micelles and are therefore transported to the sites of absorption in the same way as fatty acids and monoglycerides.

3 *Intracellular events.* Most short- and medium-chain fatty acids (12 carbon atoms or less in length) pass through the mucosal cell and enter the portal plasma. Long-chain fatty acids, monoglycerides and cholesterol are re-esterified within the mucosal cell and then incorporated into lipoprotein particles, which are then transported out of the cell into the lacteals. The spatial orientation of these particles is analogous to the micelle; thus the lipid moiety is carried within a hydrophobic core, which is surrounded by a hydrophilic membrane consisting of protein, phospholipid and free cholesterol (chylomicrons).

4 *Absorption of fat soluble vitamins.* Vitamin A esters are hydrolysed by pancreatic retinyl hydrolase. It is not yet established whether luminal hydrolysis of other fat-soluble vitamins is an important absorptive step. The fat-soluble vitamins are carried to the cell surface in mixed micelles. Once in the cell they are incorporated into chylomicrons and transported out of the cell into the lymph.

Applications to enteral nutrition

It follows from the above discussion that an adequate supply of pancreatic lipase and bile acids, together with an adequately functioning absorptive surface area, are essential for normal triglyceride assimilation. Diets containing triglycerides as an energy source should therefore not be used in patients with severe exocrine pancreatic insufficiency, or cholestatic jaundice; in patients with severe intestinal mucosal abnormalities; or in those with extensive gut resections. Claims have been made that medium chain triglycerides are assimilated in the absence of pancreatic lipase and bile acids. In fact the evidence that medium-chain triglycerides are assimilated without prior hydrolysis or micellar solubilisation is far from convincing. It is probable that in the absence of pancreatic lipase some of the medium chain triglycerides may be hydrolysed by pharyngeal lipase, and that some uptake of medium chain fatty acids occurs without micellar solubilisation. On a molecule to molecule basis, therefore, it is probable that more medium chain than long chain triglycerides will be absorbed in patients with reduced luminal lipase and bile salt concentrations. In these circumstances, the use of enteric diets containing medium chain triglycerides as the lipid energy source would be preferable to those containing triglycerides.

Carbohydrate absorption

Starch, sucrose and lactose are the main carbohydrates ingested by man (Table 7.3). Starch (Fig. 7.3) is a polysaccharide composed of glucose molecules in long chains, either with branching points (amylopectin) or without branching points (amylose). Glucose molecules in the straight chains are formed by $\alpha1–4$ linkages, whereas the branching points are created by $\alpha1–6$ linkages. Starch is rapidly hydrolysed in the lumen of the duodenum by pancreatic and salivary α-amylases (Fig. 7.3). These enzymes split only internal $\alpha1–4$ linkages, so the luminal products of starch hydrolysis consist of a mixture of $\alpha1–4$ linked glucose oligosaccharides containing between 4 and 10 glucose molecules, α-limit dextrins ($\alpha1–4$ and $\alpha1–6$ linkages), maltotriose and maltose. Lactose and sucrose are not hydrolysed by α-amylase. The products of luminal starch digestion and the two other disaccharides lactose and sucrose are hydrolysed by brush border oligosaccharidases to their constituent monosaccharides, which are then absorbed by sodium and energy-dependent carrier-mediated transport systems situated on the luminal surface of the microvillous membrane.

Table 7.3 Average daily carbohydrate intake for an adult human subject.

	Intake (g)	% of total
Polysacchardies		
Starch	200	64
Glycogen	1	0·5
Disaccharides		
Sucrose	80	26
Lactose	20	6.5
Monosaccharide		
Fructose	10	3

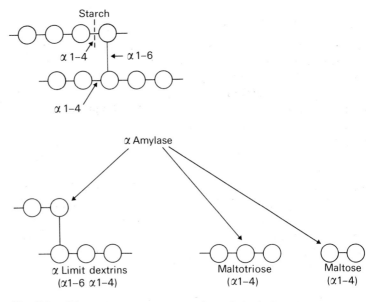

Fig. 7.3 Schematic representation of starch hydrolysis by pancreatic α-amylase. Alpha-amylase hydrolyses the α1–4 linkages of the starch molecule, and the products of hydrolysis are α-linked dextrins maltotriose and maltose.

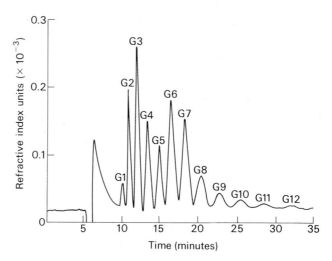

Fig. 7.4 High performance liquid chromatogram of a corn starch hydrosylate. G1 refers to glucose present as free glucose, G2 refers to glucose present as maltose, G3 as maltotriose, etc. Approximately 50% of total glucose present as higher molecular weight polymers not shown in this figure.

Although some manufacturers claim that the carbohydrate energy source of their diets consists of glucose polymers with an average chain length of five glucose molecules, our recent gel permeation chromatographic analysis shows that this is an over-simplification of the true picture. Thus Caloreen (Roussel Laboratories, Wembley Park, Middlesex), a widely used glucose polymer energy source, comprises a wide range of glucose polymers (Fig. 7.4). Recent studies in our laboratory have highlighted the differential handling of the high (>10 glucose molecules) and low (<10 glucose molecules) molecular weight fractions of corn starch hydrolysates by the human small intestine in the absence of luminal α-amylase; the lower molecular weight fractions being absorbed faster than the high molecular weight fractions [4]. The finding that maltose and maltotriose, as well as a purified low molecular weight polymer fraction containing between 5 and 7 glucose molecules all exert a kinetic advantage (on an equimolar basis, glucose absorbed faster from the oligosaccharides than from a free glucose mixture) on glucose transport [5], stimulated us to examine the absorptive properties of a complete amylase hydrolysate of corn starch which simulates the end-products of luminal starch digestion. This material also conferred a kinetic advantage on glucose absorption [4], and our most recent studies also show that a complete amylase hydrolysate of a purified high MW polymer fraction likewise confers a kinetic advantage on glucose transport [6]. The results of these studies strongly suggest that the energy content of enteric diets could be increased while at the same time reducing osmolality without there being a deleterious effect on absorptive properties if conventional carbohydrate energy sources are replaced by purified high MW glucose polymers [6].

Inherited brush border lactase deficiency is fairly common, occurring in about 6% of English people, in 20% or so of non-Caucasian Europeans and in nearly 100% of adults in many Asian and African ethnic groups [7]. A number of milk-protein-based enteric feeds contain quite large quantities of lactose, and its has been suggested that the use of these diets in patients with lactase deficiency will predispose them to diarrhoea [8]. Due to the fact that in the normal clinical setting there is very little evidence of a direct relationship between abdominal symptoms following lactose ingestion and brush border lactase levels [9] we have doubted the above claims and have recently performed a controlled clinical trial to investigate the role of lactose-containing diets on the incidence of enteral-feeding-associated diarrhoea. In fact our data show that the occurrence of diarrhoea is quite unrelated to the presence or absence of lactose in the diet, even in patients with lactase deficiency [10]. There seems no reason therefore to advocate the use of lactose free enteral diets in preference to lactose-containing diets, even in patients suspected of having lactase deficiency.

Protein absorption

The normal daily ingestion of dietary protein is usually 70–100 g, and 35–130 g of endogenous protein are secreted into the gut lumen daily [3, 11]. Absorption of dietary and endogenous protein is very efficient as the healthy adult only excretes 1–2 g of faecal nitrogen per day.

Intraluminal digestion

Protein is hydrolysed to large polypeptides by the pepsins secreted by the gastric mucosa. The large polypeptides enter the duodenum, where they are further hydrolysed by the concerted action of the different pancreatic proteolytic enzymes, namely trypsin, chymotrypsin, carboxypeptidase A and B, and elastase.

The products of luminal protein digestion consist of a mixture of free amino acids and small peptides containing 2–6 amino acid units [12]. Until recently it was believed that dietary protein required complete hydrolysis in the gut lumen or at the surface of the cell to free amino acids before absorption took place. The latest evidence, however, indicates that unhydrolysed di- and tripeptides are also absorbed from the small intestine [3, 12–14]. In man di- and tripeptides are absorbed by carrier-mediated transport systems that are independent of the group-specific free amino acid transport systems [3, 12–14].

Intestinal perfusion experiments with partial enzymic hydrolysates of whole protein which were prepared to simulate the normal products of luminal protein digestion suggest that peptide transport is likely to be quantitatively of greater significance when compared with free amino acid transport [15–17].

In the early experiments performed in man using model peptides, a consistent finding was that amino acid residues were absorbed faster when presented to the jejunal mucosa in the form of di- and tripeptides rather than in the free form [18–20]. This so called 'kinetic advantage' conferred by peptides on uptake of amino acids was also evident when absorption of amino acid residues was compared from partial enzymic hydrolysates of whole protein and their respective equimolar free amino acid mixtures [15–17]. Fig. 7.5 shows the result of one such experiment in which a partial papain hydrolysate of a casein–

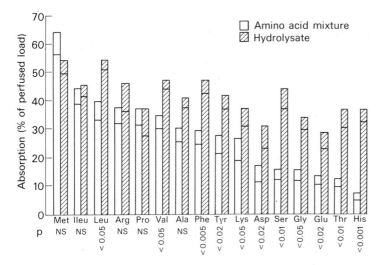

Fig. 7.5 Absorption of individual amino acid from an amino acid mixture simulating lactalbumin and lactalbumin hydrosylate. The total height of each column represents the mean value (N = 6) and 1 SE is shown as a transverse line across the column. Open columns = amino acid mixture; shaded = lactalbumin hydrosylate. NS = not significant.

soy–lactalbumin protein blend conferred a kinetic advantage on absorption of 13 of its 15 amino acid residues [21]. Thus 13 amino acid residues were absorbed significantly faster from the protein hydrolysate than from its free amino acid mixture and total absorption of infused α-amino acid nitrogen was significantly greater from the hydrolysate than from the free amino acid mixture.

Applications to enteral nutrition

Pancreatic proteolytic enzymes are secreted into the lumen of the upper small intestine in large quantities, and it is probable that in the presence of normal intestinal function up to 90% impairment of exocrine pancreatic function has to occur before luminal hydrolysis acts as a limiting step in the assimilation of amino acids from whole protein [22]. Accordingly, there seems every reason to believe that the vast majority of patients requiring enteral nutrition can be fed with an enteric diet containing whole protein as the nitrogen source. Patients with severe exocrine pancreatic insufficiency and patients with the short bowel syndrome, in whom uptake of nitrogen is limited by impaired luminal hydrolysis, require feeding with a predigested nitrogen source, preferably in the form in which amino acids are optimally absorbed. At the time the first chemically defined 'elemental' diets were formulated it was generally believed that the products of luminal protein digestion were absorbed as free amino acids, and in the light of this thinking free amino acid mixtures were used as the nitrogen source. Since subsequent research shows that not only are the products of luminal protein digestion absorbed in the form of oligopeptides, but also that peptides confer a kinetic advantage on amino acid uptake, there seems every reason to believe that when a predigested nitrogen source is required, oligopeptides rather than free amino acids should be used. The substitution of the free amino acid nitrogen sources by oligopeptides will have the added effect of lowering the osmolality of the diet, and it should be appreciated that the main advantages of a peptide versus free amino acid nitrogen source are likely to be the beneficial effects on osmolality, cost and taste rather than nutritional benefits.

Absorption of water and electrolytes

Table 7.4 lists the approximate values of water and electrolytes that are handled by the normal gut in a 24 hour period. As can be seen above, water and electrolytes entering the intestine are derived mainly from gut secretions and not from the diet. Negligible absorption takes place in the stomach. There is considerable movement of water and electrolytes into the lumen of the duodenum in response to osmotic and concentration gradients, and the early work of Fordtran and colleagues suggested that by the time the upper jejunum is reached the bulk phase of intestinal contents is isotonic [23]. The most recent studies using hypertonic liquid test meals indicate, however, that the bulk phase of jejunal luminal contents may remain somewhat

Table 7.4   Approximate mean quantities of water and electrolytes handled by the gut in 24 hours by normal subjects.

	Water (ml)	Sodium (mEq)	Chloride (mEq)	Potassium (mEq)
Input				
Diet	1500	150	150	80
Gut secretions	7500	1000	750	40
Total	9000	1150	900	120
Absorption				
Small intestine	7500	950	800	110
Colon	1350	195	97	−3
Output				
Stools	150	5	3	12

hypertonic compared to plasma [24]. The jejunum has a very limited capacity to absorb sodium and chloride from isotonic saline solutions [25, 26]. Recent experiments, however, show that the end-products of carbohydrate [25] and protein digestion [17, 26], as well as bicarbonate ions [27], have a powerful stimulatory effect on water and electrolyte absorption in the human jejunum.

In contrast to the jejunum, ileal and colonic absorption of sodium and water occurs independently of absorption of carbohydrate and protein digestion products. In these regions of the intestine sodium is transported against a concentration and electrical gradient (active transport) [28], and chloride is absorbed against a concentration gradient but down an electrical gradient. Furthermore, chloride ions are absorbed more avidly than sodium ions and against larger concentration gradients. It has been proposed that anionic and cationic exchange systems operate independently of each other [29], and it is assumed that water absorption follows sodium transport passively.

Applications to enteral nutrition

The important function of the duodenum in attempting to render gastric contents isotonic by the time the jejunum is reached, has considerable relevance to enteral nutrition. The rapid infusion of hypertonic enteric diets will result in considerable fluxes of water and electrolytes into the lumen of the duodenum, thereby presenting the small intestine with large loads of water and electrolytes for absorption. It is the inability of the small intestine, especially when diseased, to assimilate such large quantities of fluid and electrolytes that is thought to be one of the underlying causes for the diarrhoea that occurs during enteral feeding. Attempts can be made to circumvent this problem by reducing the osmotic load presented to the duodenum during feeding. This can be done by administering dilute diets, particularly at the start of treatment, and by infusing the diets continuously over a 24 hour period. Although the reasons for it are not completely understood, patients appear to be able to adapt to increasingly hypertonic loads over a 3–5 day period, so that the strength of the diets may be increased incrementally over this period, and full strength feeding is usually possible by days 3–5.

DIET FORMULATION

1   *Diets for patients with normal gastrointestinal function.* Patients with normal gastrointestinal function are capable of assimilating whole protein and unhydrolysed triglyceride. Enteric diets for

these patients (Table 7.5) should therefore contain whole protein as the nitrogen source and triglycerides and carbohydrates as the energy source. As our recent physiological studies indicate [8] that high molecular weight glucose polymers (>10 glucose units) are efficiently assimilated by the normal human jejunum in the absence of amylase, the carbohydrate component of the energy source could more ideally consist of purified high molecular weight glucose polymers rather than the more widely used heterogeneous glucose polymer mixtures derived from the *in vitro* hydrolysis of starch that contain low, as well as high, molecular weight polymers.

In our experience the majority of patients requiring enteral nutrition have nitrogen requirements in the range 9–15 g/24 hr, so we believe that the non-protein energy to nitrogen ratio of these diets should be in the region of 150–200:1. As the onset of diarrhoea during enteric feeding is likely to be due, at least in part, to intolerance of the high osmotic loads presented to the duodenum during administration, there is every reason to believe that these diets should be isotonic with plasma and therefore have an osmolality in the range of 285–300 mosmol/kg. This can be achieved without diluting the diet if the high molecular weight glucose polymers are used instead of low molecular weight material. Finally the enteric diets for those patients with normal gastrointestinal function should contain sufficient electrolyte, trace elements and vitamins to satisfy nutritional requirements.

2 *Diets for patients with impaired gastrointestinal function.* In a small group of patients, nutrient assimilation may be impaired on account of insufficient luminal nutrient hydrolysis or because the functional absorptive capacity of the intestine is so reduced as not to be able to cope with the quantities of nutrients presented to it for absorption. In these circumstances it follows that nutrients should be presented to the gut in a predigested form, and indeed to

Table 7.5 Composition of ideal standard enteric diet.

Nitrogen source	Whole protein
Energy source	Carbohydrate (65%)—high MW glucose polymers
	Fat (35%)—triglycerides
Non-protein energy nitrogen ratio (kcal/g)	150–200:1
Electrolytes	
Minerals	
Vitamins	
Osmolality	285–300 mosmol/kg

ensure that the maximal possible absorption is achieved the predigested nutrients should ideally be presented in the form in which they are absorbed fastest in the normal clinical setting.

Conditions in which luminal nutrient hydrolysis is severely impaired include severe exocrine pancreatic insufficiency, obstructive jaundice and the short bowel syndrome. The functional absorptive capacity of the intestine may be severely reduced in the short bowel syndrome and in clinical conditions characterized by a severe and extensive mucosal lesion (coeliac disease, severe Crohn's disease). These then become the indications for the use of predigested diets (Table 7.6). The old term 'elemental diet' is a misnomer. Used initially to describe the early free amino acid- and glucose-containing diets, it was later used to describe all the other diets containing predigested nutrients that were far from 'elemental' in design.

The use of 'elemental' diets has been advocated in a variety of clinical conditions [30] including the management of gastrointestinal fistulae, inflammatory bowel disease, the nutritional management of patients with gastrointestinal cancer and those with severe maldigestion and malabsorption and, finally, their use as a means of pre-operative bowel preparation has also been suggested. In a brilliant exposé of the myths surrounding the indications and uses of 'elemental' diets, Koretz and Meyer [31] point out that there is very little controlled data to support any of these claims. In our unit, we have just shown [32] that there is no evidence for the superiority of 'elemental' over polymeric diets containing whole protein as the nitrogen source in the management of malnourished patients with normal gastrointestinal

Table 7.6 Indications for use of predigested 'elemental' diets.

1	Impaired luminal nutrient ingestion	
	Severe exocrine pancreatic insufficiency	Total pancreatectomy
		Carcinoma of pancreas
		Severe chronic pancreatitis
	Short bowel syndrome	Intestinal resections
		Intestinal fistulae
2	Reduced functional absorptive capacity	Intestinal resections
		Intestinal fistulae
		Severe untreated coeliac disease
		Severe active Crohn's disease*

*rare

function, an observation that was also noted during an investigation of the efficacy of 'elemental' and polymeric diets in unconscious patients with head injury [33].

As mentioned above the nitrogen source of these predigested diets should, in the light of our current knowledge, consist of oligopeptides rather than free amino acids. Partial enzymic hydrolysates of whole protein constitute the most suitable peptide-based nitrogen source, although the optimum starter protein, hydrolysis procedure and peptide chain length have yet to be defined. As our intestinal perfusion studies indicate the purified high molecular weight polymers are assimilated in the absence of luminal amylase activity [6] these should probably constitute the carbohydrate fraction of the energy source.

Since these diets are properly indicated in conditions in which luminal fat digestion is impaired, they should not contain large amounts of triglyceride-based energy source. As mentioned previously, it is not clear as to whether large quantities of medium-chain triglycerides are absorbed in the absence of luminal hydrolysis, so MCTs should probably not be included in these diets. The diets should contain at least 4% of their total energy content as linoleic acid, however, to prevent the development of essential fatty acid deficiency that has been described during long term Vivonex (Eaton Laboratories, Woking, Surrey) treatment.

By virtue of the nature of the nitrogen source, and the fact that the energy source of the ideal elemental diet will be made up predominantly of carbohydrate, the osmolality will be higher than the standard enteric diets. The ideal elemental diet should, of course, contain sufficient electrolytes, trace elements and vitamins to satisfy the requirements of the average malnourished patient.

ENTERAL DIETS CURRENTLY AVAILABLE

Hospital tube feeds

Before the recent resurgence of interest in enteral nutrition, those patients with normal gastrointestinal function who did receive nutritional support were fed with tube feeds prepared in the hospital dietetic department. The composition of a typical diet that used to be prepared in our dietetic department is shown in Table 7.7. It is dubious whether the patient's electrolyte, trace element and vitamin requirements are properly satisfied during prolonged feeding, and the osmolality is quite high. Although these tube feeds are cheap, the preparation of large quantities places a significant burden on the workload of the dietetic department, which is the major reason why they are not routinely used in our hospital. Care should be taken to ensure that the diets are prepared under reasonably sterile conditions, as problems with infection have been well documented [34, 35] and there is now controlled data to show that the incidence of diarrhoea is higher when 'home brew', rather than commercial diets, are used for enteral feeding [36].

Proprietary polymeric enteric diets

Some of the more widely used proprietary polymeric diets are listed in Table 7.8. All are low-residue and all contain whole protein. The price of the different diets varies, even when calculated per gram of nitrogen. All but Isocal are said to be palatable and thus suitable for oral supplementation. In our experience, though, patient-acceptance is not as good as the manufacturers claim.

There are considerable variations in the non-nitrogen calorie to nitrogen ratios of the different diets. With the exception Clinifeed-Iso, the ratios are less than 200:1, and consequently the other diets may require supplementation with a carbohydrate

Table 7.7 Typical hospital tube feed.

Ingredients	*Elements*
1000 ml milk	Sodium 40 mmol
120 g Complan	Potassium 67 mmol
50 g Caloreen	Calcium 2076 mg
50 ml corn oil	Phosphorus 950 mg
0.6 ml Abidec	Magnesium 140 mg
Nutrient content	*Vitamins*
Nitrogen 9.28 g	A 5670 IU
Fat 106 g (954 kcal)	D 466 IU
Carbohydrate 184 g (736 kcal)	Thiamine 2.7 mg
	Riboflavin 3.1 mg
Non-protein energy nitrogen ratio	Pyridoxine 1.4 mg
182:1	Nicotinic acid 15 mg
Recommended supplements	*Ingredients*
Folicin 2 tablets daily	Folic acid 5 mg,
	copper sulphate 5 mg,
	manganese sulphate 5 mg,
	ferrous sulphate 340 mg
	sulphate 340 mg
Zincomed 1 capsule daily	Zinc sulphate 220 mg
Vitamin B12 1000 μg i.m. monthly	

energy source. Caloreen and Maxijul are two rather similar soluble glucose polymer mixtures that can be used as energy supplements. All but Clinifeed-400 are lactose-free. The osmolality of these diets ranged from 250 mosmol/kg for Triosorbon to 450 mosmol/kg for Ensure. With the exception of Triosorbon all contain long-chain triglycerides, and these contribute variously to the total energy content of the diets. Triosorbon contains medium-chain triglycerides (MCT) and not long-chain triglycerides and may be better handled by patients with obstructive jaundice who have normal luminal concentrations of amylase and proteolytic enzymes, but reduced luminal bile salt concentrations, due to obstruction of bile outflow.

With the exception of the above comments pertaining to Triosorbon, there is no hard clinical evidence that any single diet listed in Table 7.8 has any clinical or significant advantage over the others [33].

Chemically defined 'elemental' diets

Some of the more widely-used diets currently available in the U K are shown in Table 7.9. Vivonex Standard and Vivonex High Nitrogen (Eaton) are the two diets that contain free amino acids as their nitrogen source. On account of this they are hypertonic, unpalatable and expensive. Flexical (Mead Johnson) was the first predigested 'elemental diet' to contain a so-called 'peptide'-based nitrogen source. The exact profile of the nitrogen source in respect of peptide chain length and proportions of peptide-bound and free amino acid residues is, however, not known. This diet is also expensive and unpalatable. Nutranel is probably the predi-

Table 7.8 Proprietary polymeric enteral diets, all of which have a whole protein nitrogen source.

Diet	Flavouring necessary	Presentation	Osmolality mosmol/kg	Non-protein energy/Nitrogen ratio (kcal/gN)
Build up (Carnation)	No	Powder	575	100
Clinifeed 400 (Roussel)	No	Liquid	426	142
Clinifeed Favour (Roussel)	No	Liquid	403	142
Clinifeed Iso (Roussel)	No	Liquid	321	200
Ensure (Abbott)	No	Liquid	430	154
Isocal (Mead Johnson)	Yes	Liquid	350	170
Nutrauxil (Kabivitrum)	No	Liquid	386	140
Trisorbon (BDH)	No	Powder	400	130

gested diet of choice in the UK; it is cheaper than the other two diets, contains a well-balanced peptide-based nitrogen source and is relatively palatable.

Routes of administration

Oral feeding

When the patient is able to swallow, but still unable to eat normal food (e.g. because of an oesophageal stricture), a liquid diet can be provided from any hospital diet kitchen. The large volume of fluid required to liquidise whole food may make this type of supplement unacceptable to some patients.

The palatable standard enteric diets and the elemental diets listed in Tables 7.8 and 7.9 are suitable for oral feeding, both as a

Table 7.9 Proprietary chemically defined 'elemental' diets.

Diet	Flavouring necessary	Nitrogen source	Presentation	Osmolality mosmol/kg	Non-protein energy/ nitrogen ratio (kcal/gN)
Flexical (Mead Johnson)	Yes	Oligopeptides/ Free amino acids	Powder	580	256
Nutranel (Roussel)	Yes	Oligopeptides	Powder	550	131
Survimed	No	Oligopeptides	Powder	456	152
Vivonex HN (Eaton)	Yes	Free amino acids	Powder	830	121

means of supplementing an inadequate intake of normal food and as the sole means of nutritional support. As stated above, elemental diets should only be used in preference to the standard enteric diets if positive indications for their use (Table 7.6) are present.

If it is planned to use the proprietary enteric diets as the sole means of nutritional support, we prefer to administer the diets via a nasogastric tube, because we find it easier to precisely document and control intake. Another reason is that the patients find that most of the diets are not as palatable as the manufacturers claim and excessive nursing time is taken up cajoling patients to ingest the desired quantities.

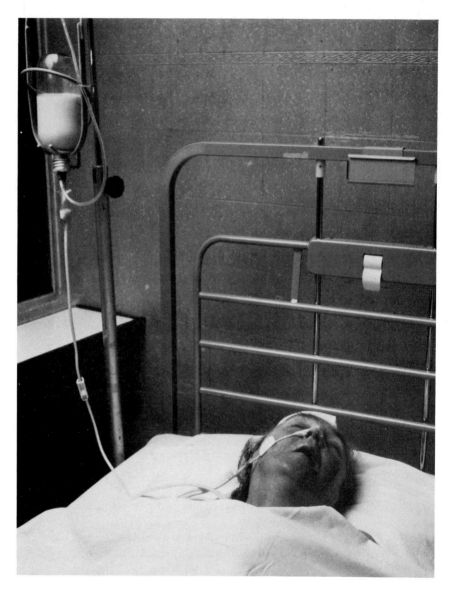

Fig. 7.6 Enteral feeding of a patient following neurosurgery. Patient is intubated nasogastrically with a fine bore feeding tube, and receiving an enteral diet by constant gravity infusion from a 500 ml glass container via a standard giving set.

Patients who cannot swallow, or who will not tolerate oral feeding, can be fed via a nasogastric tube.

The time-honoured method of tube feeding has been to place a large-bore Ryles tube into the stomach and intermittently to instil up to 200 ml liquid feed, having first aspirated the gastric residue. This method is probably responsible for the poor reputation of enteral feeding, as the incidence of side-effects, namely diarrhoea, aspiration pneumonia and oesophageal ulceration, has been unacceptably high.

Major new developments have taken place in this field and most of these problems have now been circumvented. Enteric feeds (Fig. 7.6) can be administered from containers by gravity infusion via narrow-bore polyvinyl chloride (PVC), erythrothane or silicone feeding tubes, most of which are inserted, with the aid of an introducer, into the stomach. These fine-bore tubes are more comfortable than the older wider bore tubes and their use has not so far been associated with oesophageal erosions, ulcers or strictures. Although easy to pass, the final position should be checked radiologically or by insufflating 5 ml air and auscultating over the epigastrium to ensure that the feeding tube has been positioned in the stomach (Fig. 7.7) and not the bronchial tree.

In a small proportion of patients, usually those with carcinoma of the oesophagus or cardia of the stomach, intubation using standard techniques proves impossible. In some of these, the feeding tube can be passed into the stomach under direct endoscopic control.

Types of feeding tubes. As Fig. 7.8 shows, there are now a large number of fine-bore feeding tubes on the market. Broadly speaking there are the simple unweighted tubes (we use the 1 mm diameter Clinifeeding system I tube introduced with a wire introducer marketed by Roussel Laboratories) or feeding tubes with mercury-weighted tips. In our experience, in routine clinical use, the more expensive mercury-weighted tubes offer few advantages over the simple unweighted and open-ended feeding tubes. There are 3 clinical areas, however, where we have noted distinct advantages [37].

1   Nasogastric intubation of patients already intubated with an endotracheal tube.
2   Intubation of patients with oesophageal strictures in whom endoscopic intubation with unweighted tubes has failed.
3   Nasoenteric feeding (see below).

Endoscopic tube placement. Although nasogastric tube placement usually presents few problems, difficulties do arise when attempts are made to perform nasogastric intubation in patients with oesophageal strictures, and nasoenteric intubation of those with gastric atony. In the first group of patients, irrespective of whether the stricture is malignant or benign, intubation is usually required either during diagnostic endoscopy or immediately following endoscopic dilatation. In the second group, despite claims to the contrary [38, 39], feeding tubes rarely pass through the pylorus spontaneously, and have to be placed in the jejunum or duodenum at endoscopy.

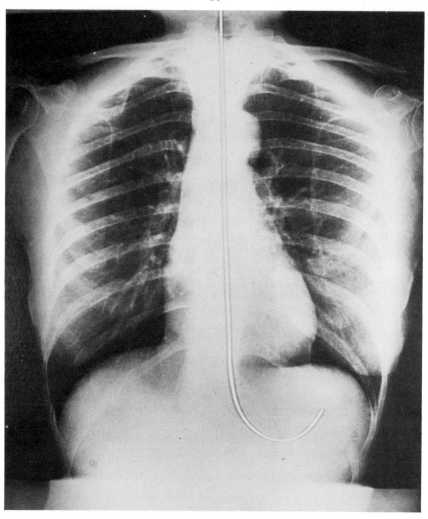

Fig. 7.7 X-ray of the chest and upper abdomen showing fine bore nasogastric feeding tube correctly positioned below the diaphragm and in the fundus of the stomach. For clarity of presentation the outline of the tube has been enhanced by a medical artist.

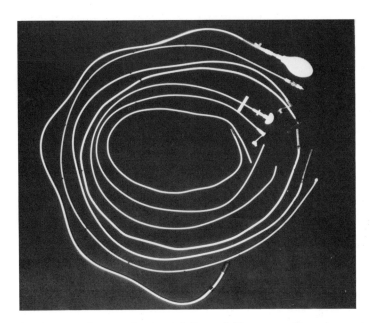

Fig. 7.8 A selection of commercially available nasogastric and nasoen-teric feeding tubes. From inside to outside: (1) Clinifeeding System 1 (Roussel Laboratories; PVC, 70 cm, int. diam 1 mm); (2) Entri nasogastric feeding tube (Biosearch; Erythrothane, 81 cm, no. 6 French); (3) Prima enteral feeding tube (Portex; PVC, 85 cm, 1.1 mm); (4) Hydromer-Dobbhoff enteric feeding tube (Biosearch; Erythrothane, 109 cm, no. 8 French); (5) Entriflex nasogastric feeding tube (Biosearch; Erythrothane, 91 cm, no. 8 French); (6) Enteral feeding tube (SHS; Silicone, 125 cm, no. 7 French); (7) Duo Tube enteral feeding unit (Argyle; Silicone, 102 cm, no. 8 French).

Atkinson and co-workers [40] described a technique of endoscopic tube placement requiring the passage of an endo-scope, oral passage of the feeding tube, which is subsequently grasped by endoscopic biopsy forceps and correctly positioned, with the final nasal exit position being achieved by passing a Ryles tube and retrogradely passing the feeding tube up it.

We have encountered a number of problems with this technique which include the inability to insufflate air during endoscopy, difficulty in grasping and holding the feeding tube and poor patient tolerance, particularly if the procedure becomes time consuming. The following is a description of the technique used in our unit [41].

After applying topical anaesthesia to the oropharynx, a fine-bore nasogastric feeding tube is passed with the aid of an internal stiffening wire until the distal end is visible in the oropharynx. The internal stiffening wire is then removed and the tube is easily grasped with McGill forceps and brought out through the mouth (Fig. 7.9). The distal 5–10 cm of tube is inserted up the biopsy channel of a GIFP (Olympus) endoscope. The tube makes a snug but not airtight fit, thus permitting air insufflation without allowing the tube to slip out, even during normal endoscopic manoeuvres. The endoscope with attached tube, which impedes neither vision or manoeuvrability, is passed until the desired position is reached. The feeding tube is then voided by passing the biopsy forceps down the channel and pushing it out. If required, tissue biopsy or brushings can now be performed normally and the endoscope then removed, leaving the feeding tube *in situ.*

Nasoenteric feeding. In certain patients with neurological disorders of swallowing mechanism (e.g. motorneurone disease, pseudobulbar palsy) or gastric atony, regurgitation or aspiration of enteric feeds administered nasogastrically necessitates the cessation of nasogastric feeding. Theoretically, these side-effects should be circumvented by direct duodenal or jejunal feeding. In most cases, we have found it difficult to directly intubate the duodenum with any of the currently available simple or mercury-weighted tubes, and have been unable to substantiate earlier claims [37, 38] that simple or mercury-tipped feeding tubes spontaneously pass through the pylorus, particularly if there is

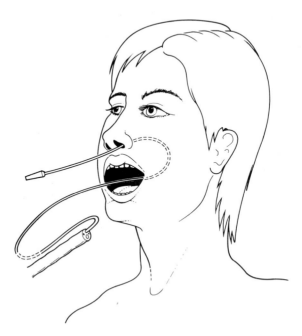

Fig. 7.9 Arrangement of a fine bore nasogastric feeding tube prior to distal endoscopic positioning.

co-existing gastric atony. In these circumstances we use an endoscopic method of tube placement in which a 3 mm external (1.8 mm internal) diameter tube with an integral 3 g mercury tip of smaller external diameter (Nutriflex, Biosearch) is used. The tube is passed into the stomach in the normal manner and the stiffener wire partially removed. The tube is then grasped with the endoscopic biopsy forceps and after complete removal of the stiffening wire the feeding tube is pushed forward in front of the endoscope to the desired position in the duodenum.

Early post-operative nasoenteral feeding. The recognition that small bowel function returns earlier on in the post-operative period than gastric function [42, 43] has lead to the concept of early post-operative enteral feeding via a fine needle catheter jejunostomy or via nasoenteric tubes positioned at the time of laparotomy [44, 45]. On theoretical grounds, this would appear to represent an ideal means of providing nutritional support in the early post-operative period, although the data is far from clear in respect of clinical advantages [45]. In most of the published studies 'elemental' rather than polymeric diets were used (for which there appears to be little rationale) and in the one controlled study [44] which claims advantages, the only possible benefit (and a questionable one at that) that seems actually to have accrued in the treatment group was that the patients were discharged from hospital sooner than those not receiving nutritional support.

Administration techniques

As mentioned previously, enteric diets are best administered from feed reservoirs via a giving set and feeding tube directly into the stomach, duodenum or jejunum (Fig. 7.6). There has been a recent proliferation of delivery systems (Fig. 7.10), and debate exists as to the ideal volume of the feed reservoirs. A recent study [35] indicates that feeds which are mixed in the diet kitchen are subject to significant bacterial contamination (e.g. preparation of standard tube feeds or energy supplementation of other feeds). During administration, bacterial multiplication occurs, so those diets, if used, should not be prepared in volumes of more than 0.5 litres. No significant bacterial contamination of pre-sterilised enteral feeds appears to occur during filling of reservoirs, so if these diets are followed up to 2 litre volume reservoirs can be used.

Enteral feeding pumps

In our unit all diets are administered continuously over 24 hours, as a means of reducing the incidence of gastrointestinal side-effects (see below). In a prospective study [46] over 85% of 80 patients were fed successfully when the diets were administered by simple gravity infusion using the giving-set clamp to control the infusion rate. Clearly, therefore, one does not have to advocate the routine use of an enteral feeding pump. The use of a pump was, however, shown to be beneficial in patients with impaired gastrointestinal function who developed diarrhoea during enteral feeding and a saving of up to 30 minutes nursing time per patient per day can be achieved if diets are administered using an enteral feeding pump.

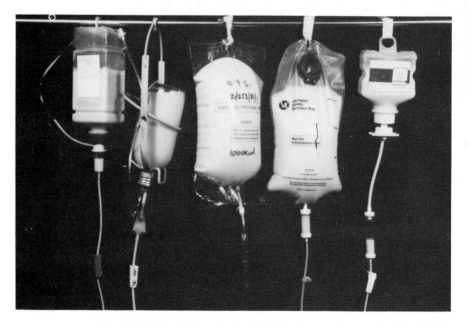

Fig. 7.10 A selection of enteral feeding bags and reservoirs. From left to right: (1) Roussel Clinifeeding System 3 (1.3 l); (2) Re-useable DHSS Winchester container (0.5 l); (3) Express enteral feeding bag (2 l); (4) Viomedex enteral feeding bag (1.5 l); (5) Boots Flow Fusor enteral feeding bottle (0.5 l).

Prescribing the regime

As the aim of nutritional support is, wherever possible, to place patients in positive nitrogen balance, the first aim of any treatment programme is to determine nitrogen losses. Ideally, nitrogen losses in urine, faeces and any ostomy effluent should be accurately measured. Available methods for measuring the nitrogen content of biological fluids are time-consuming and costly. Recent work [47, 48] has shown that nitrogen losses can be more simply calculated from measurements of 24 hour urinary urea excretion—urea being the major end-product of endogenous protein metabolism. Thus:

Nitrogen loss

$$(\text{g}/24\text{ hrs}) = \text{urinary urea (mmol}/24\text{ hrs} \times 0.028) + 2$$

where the factor of 2 represents non-urinary nitrogen excretion.

Modifications to this formula are required if the blood urea is high or rising or the patient has proteinuria [49] and the formula cannot be used for patients with protein-losing enteropathies, or in patients who have excessive nitrogen losses in fistulae or ostomy effluents.

Positive nitrogen balance can only be achieved if nitrogen intake exceeds output, and as a rule of thumb we base our regime on a nitrogen intake of approximately 3–5 g N in excess of output. As it is difficult to increase muscle mass and body weight in immobilised patients, aggressive physiotherapy and exercising is encouraged whenever possible.

Use of starter regimes

Upper abdominal symptoms including distension, discomfort and colicky pains, as well as diarrhoea, are said to frequently occur if full-strength enteric feeding regimes are introduced too quickly [50]. The pathogenesis of these side-effects is most likely related to the movement of fluid and electrolytes into the lumen of the upper small intestine in response to the high osmotic load of solute presented to the mucosa during diet administration. It is generally believed that the incidence of these side-effects can be minimised by gradually introducing full-strength enteric feeds over a 3–4 day period by means of 'starter regimes'. A typical such regime is summarised in Table 7.10.

Table 7.10 Starter regimes.

Day	Strength	Volume (litres)
Normal gastrointestinal function		
1	Half	2
2	Three-quarter	2
3	Full	2
4	Exact composition modified according to nitrogen balance studies conducted over previous 3 days	
Impaired gastrointestinal function		
1	Quarter	1–1.5
	Strength and volume should be cautiously increased over 5–7 days	

In reality, it was probably the outmoded technique of bolus feeding that gave rise to the high incidence of gastrointestinal side-effects. Currently we are re-examining the need for starter regimes in patients who are fed continuously over 24 hours with diets that have osmolalities closely isotonic with plasma.

Success of enteral feeding

The true benefits of enteral feeding, as with other forms of nutritional support, have been hard to define scientifically. In our judgement, however, considerable benefits to the patients have occurred despite the lack of objective proof. We have found, for example, that the median period of enteral feeding in two controlled clinical trials [10, 32] is 11 and 15 days respectively, after which patients have usually been able to return to a normal diet. We have not, however, been able to show marked improvement in the nutritional parameters in this time, and contrary to initial expectations the treatment groups as a whole have not always been placed in overall positive nitrogen balance [10, 32]. There are a number of reasons for this, which include the ease with which the new narrow-bore feeding tubes may be regurgitated or removed by the patient, poor feeding technique (in which the diet is infused too slowly), the inherent difficulties of converting the stressed catabolic patient into positive nitrogen balance, the onset of side-effects such as vomiting and diarrhoea, and the need for some patients undergoing investigation to fast.

COMPLICATIONS OF ENTERAL NUTRITION (Table 7.11)

Tube-related problems

Complications previously associated with larger-bore Ryles tubes, namely oesophageal erosions, haemorrhage and strictures [52], have not been reported with the fine-bore nasogastric tubes. The fine bore tube can be passed in the trachea rather than the oesophagus, especially in comatose patients, so the previously mentioned care must be taken to ensure correct positioning before enteric feeding is started. One common problem with the narrow bore feeding tube is the ease with which the tube rides up into the oesophagus, or is removed by the patient, and in our experience nearly all patients on enteric feeding regimes will require more than one intubation. Intravenous administration of an enteric feed has been reported [48], although this complication should not occur if feeding tubes and giving sets are used with reversed luers, thus ensuring that intravenous and enteral feeding systems are incompatible.

Table 7.11 Complications of enteral nutrition.

95
Enteral Feeding

Tube insertion	Metabolic complications
Oesophagitis	Hyperglycaemia
Oesophagel erosions	Hypokalaemia
Oesophageal stricture	Hypomagnesaemia
Tube misplacement	Hypocalcaemia
Tube withdrawal	Hypophosphataemia
	Low zinc levels
Regurgitation and aspiration	Low RBC folate
Gastrointestinal side-effects	Abnormalities of liver function
Diarrhoea	
Abdominal distension	Intravenous administration of
Abdominal pain	enteric feeds

Gastrointestinal side-effects

Nausea, diarrhoea, abdominal distension and pain are the commonest side-effects of enteral nutrition, occurring in up to 25% of our patients, all of whom are fed by constant gravity infusion [10, 32]. These side-effects still limit the use of enteral nutrition in a significant number of patients. The onset of abdominal distension and upper abdominal discomfort is most likely to be related to the influx of fluid and electrolytes that follows the instillation of high osmotic loads of solute into the upper small intestine during enteral feeding. The pathogenesis of the diarrhoea that develops during enteric feeding has not been so fully elucidated (see Table 7.12). Early on in most investigators' experiences the diarrhoea was often caused by the use of infected feeds [34]. Bacteriological studies show that significant bacterial contamination may occur during mixing of any type of diet in a diet kitchen [35] and clinicians are recommended to use sterilised feeds supplied in a can, as no contamination of these feeds occurs during aseptic filling of the reservoir [35].

Although not clearly understood, there is a relationship between the occurrence of diarrhoea during enteral feeding and concomitant antibiotic therapy [10]. Either intravenous or oral antibiotics appear to cause diarrhoea, although by what mechanism is not yet clear. Lactase deficiency, although often quoted as a cause of diarrhoea during enteral feeding [52], could not be implicated during a recent prospective study [10]. It is thought that many cases of diarrhoea occur because the functional absorptive capacity of the small intestine and colon cannot deal with the large volumes of fluid and electrolytes that are secreted into the lumen of the small intestine in response to the rapid ingestion of hypertonic enteric diets. Slower introduc-

Table 7.12 Postulated causes of diarrhoea and suggested remedies.

Cause	Remedy
Infected feeds	Use commercially sterilised feeds. Dilute if necessary with boiled distilled water. Add to feed reservoir in ward and not diet kitchen
Concomitant antibiotics and/or laxatives	Stop laxatives; stop antibiotics if clinically possible
Lactase deficiency	Said in the past to have been an important cause for the diarrhoea developing in non-Caucasians. No longer evidence to favour this [10]. Many will still advocate the use of lactose-free diets—we do not
Intolerance of high osmotic loads administered during feeding	Use 'starter regimes' (Table 7.10) Continuous infusion of diet over 24 hours, with or without pump-assisted infusion. Codeine phosphate 30–60 mg tds or imodium (up to 4 mg tds) may be tried

tion of full-strength feeds, as suggested in Table 7.10, and the continuous infusion of the diets over 24 hours, together with precision control of the infusion rate using a feeding pump in patients with gastrointestinal pathology [46], are practical ways in which the incidence of diarrhoea can be reduced.

Regurgitation and aspiration

Regurgitation of enteric feeds up into the oesophagus, followed on occasions by pulmonary aspiration, occurs most commonly in patients who have problems with gastric emptying and in those with neurological disease, particularly affecting the swallowing reflex. Problems with gastric emptying arise in post-operative patients, those with cerebrovascular accidents and those who have suffered recent severe trauma.

If gastric emptying is uncertain, a Ryles tube should be passed, and 60 ml of a mixture of milk and water is given hourly, with the stomach being aspirated every 4 hours. If only small amounts are aspirated enteral feeding can be commenced using up to a maximum of 2 litres of half-strength feed per 24 hrs. If the diet is well-tolerated then more concentrated feeds can be introduced, and the Ryles tube replaced with a fine-bore feeding tube. If delayed gastric emptying persists then intraduodenal feeding will have to be performed. As mentioned above, the only reliable way that a feeding tube can be positioned into the duodenum when gastric emptying is impaired is by intubating the duodenum under endoscopic control. In our experience, endoscopic tube placement is also often required in patients with neurological defects of the swallowing reflex in whom intraduodenal feeding is indicated.

Metabolic complications

Metabolic complications occur commonly during enteral feeding. Hyperglycaemia may occur during enteric feeding, caused by excessive sugar intake or insulin resistance associated with trauma and injury [51]. Initially there should be frequent urine testing for sugar, as well as measurement of blood sugar.

Electrolyte abnormalities commonly occur during enteral nutrition, and are related not only to the feeding regimes but also to the underlying medical or surgical disorder.

In one recent controlled trial [32] we found that up to half of the patients treated developed hypokalaemia and hypophospha-taemia and nearly one-third had biochemical evidence of zinc deficiency. These abnormalities highlight the need for careful monitoring and administration of supplements during enteral feeding.

Abnormalities of liver function

Abnormal liver function tests have been reported in patients receiving enteral as well as parenteral nutrition [52]. The aetiology of these changes is uncertain. Changes include elevations of alkaline phosphatase, gamma glutamyl transpeptidase and the hepatocellular enzymes, as well as occasional and mild elevations in bilirubin levels. We have been unable to confirm earlier reports that abnormalities of liver function inevitably occur during enteral nutrition, although we have quite often observed minor changes in liver function tests during enteral feeding. Thus in our clinical trial [32] up to 40% of patients develop abnormalities of their alkaline phosphatase or trans-aminases [32]. Overall we attach little significance to such changes and have never abandoned enteral feeding on account of them.

Occasionally, quite marked and persistent elevations of alka-line phosphatase occur. However, the highest levels (up to 1000 IU/l) have been observed before the start of therapy and liver biopsies performed in our unit show that rises in alkaline phosphatase are likely to be due to marked fatty infiltration of the liver, presumably related to the underlying protein calorie malnutrition. In our experience all tests return to normal after stopping enteral nutrition.

Patient monitoring

A full clinical, biochemical, haematological and immunological assessment of nutritional status should be performed before

Table 7.13   Patient monitoring in enteral nutrition.

Parameters	Before treatment	Daily	Twice weekly	Weekly
Weight	√			√
Mid triceps skin fold thickness	√			√
Arm muscle circumference	√			√
Serum albumin	√			√
Serum transferrin	√			√
Lymphocyte count	√			√
Skin tests for candida:	√			√
PPD (tuberculin)				
Streptokinase				
Streptodornase				
FBP ESR	√		√	
Serum iron	√			√
Folic acid	√			√
Vitmain B12	√			√
Prothrombin time	√			√
Blood glucose*	√	√		
Urinary glucose	√	√		
Electrolytes and urea	√		√	
Calcium	√		√	
Phosphate	√		√	
Magnesium	√		√	
Liver function tests	√			√
Zinc	√			√
24 hour urinary urea excretion† (for nitrogen balance estimations)	√	√		

* For first week only if blood glucose within normal limits and there is no glycosuria.
† It is our practice to perform daily estimations (recommended definitely for one week to estimate nitrogen requirements). Twice weekly thereafter will usually be sufficient, unless the clinical condition of patient changes.

enteral nutrition is instituted, and baseline values obtained for all other haematological and biochemical measurements. The recommendations shown in Table 7.13 are guidelines. If electrolyte or other abnormalities occur, measurements should be made at more frequent intervals. Careful monitoring is important to ensure early identification of the possible serious complications of enteral nutrition.

References

1   Borgstrom D., Dahlqvist A., Lundh G. & Sjovall J. (1957) Studies of intestinal digestion and absorption in the human. *J. Clin. Invest.* **36**, 1521.

2   Hofmann A.F. & Poley J.R. (1969) Cholestyramine treatment of diarrhoea associated with ileal resection. *New. Engl. J. Med.* **281**, 397.

3   Silk D.B.A. & Dawson A.M. (1979) Intestinal absorption of carbohydrate and protein in man. International Review of Physiology. *Gastrointestinal Physiology III* **19**, 151.

4   Jones B.J.M., Brown B.E. & Silk D.B.A. (1980) Comparison of oligosaccharide and free glucose absorption from the normal human jejunum. *Gut* **21**, A905.

5   Jones B.J.M., Brown B.E. & Silk D.B.A. (1981) Intestinal absorption of maltotriose and a maltopentose-hexose mixture in man. *Gut* **22**, A868.

6   Jones B.J.M., Brown B.E., Grimble G.K. & Silk D.B.A. (1981) The formulation of energy dense enteral feeds—the use of high molecular weight glucose polymers. *J. Parent. Ent. Nutr.* **5**, 359.

7   Neale G. (1968) The diagnosis, incidence and significance of disaccharidase deficiency in adults. *Proc. Roy. Soc. Med.* **61**, 1099.

8   McMichael H.B. (1979) Physiology of carbohydrates, electrolyte and water absorption. *Res. Clin. Forums.* **1**, 25.

9   Haverberg L., Kwon P.H. & Scrimshaw N.S. (1980) Comparative tolerance of adolescents of differing ethnic backgrounds to lactose-containing and lactose-free dairy drinks. *Am. J. Clin. Nutr.* **33**, 17.

10 Keohane P.P., Jones B.J.M. & Silk D.B.A. (1983) The role of lactose intolerance and *Clostridium difficile* infection in the pathogenesis of enteral-feeding-associated diarrhoea. *Clin. Nutr.* (in press).

11 Silk D.B.A. (1981) Peptide transport. *Clin. Sci.* **60**, 607.

12 Chen M.L., Rogers B.R. & Harper A.G. (1962) Observations on protein digestion in vivo. IV. Further observations on the gastrointestinal contents of rats fed different dietary proteins. *J. Nutr.* **76**, 235.

13 Matthews D.M. (1971) Protein absorption. *J. Clin. Pathol.* **5** (Suppl 24), 29.

14 Matthews D.M. & Adibi S.A. (1976) Peptide absorption. *Gastroenterology* **71**, 151.

15 Silk D.B.A., Marrs T.C., Addison J.M., *et al* (1973) Absorption of

amino acids from an amino acid mixture simulating casein and a tryptic hydrolysate of casein in man. *Clin. Sci. Mol. Med.* **45**, 715.

16 Silk D.B.A., Clark M.L., Marrs T. C., *et al* (1975) Jujunal absorption of an enzymic hydrolysate of casein prepared for oral administration to normal adults. *Br. Nutr.* **33**, 95.

17 Silk D.B.A., Fairclough P.D., Clark M.L., *et al* (1980) Use of a peptide rather than free amino acid nitrogen source in chemically defined 'elemental' diets. *J. Parent. Ent. Nutr.* **4**, 548.

18 Silk D.B.A., Perrett D. & Clark M.L. (1973) Intestinal transport of two dipeptides containing the same two neutral amino acids in man. *Clin. Med.* **45**, 291.

19 Silk D.B.A., Perrett D., Webb J.P.W., *et al* (1973) Tripeptide absorption in man. *Gut* **14**, 427.

20 Adibi S.A. (1971) Intestinal transport of dipeptides in man: relative importance of hydrolysis and intact absorption. *J. Clin. Invest.* **50**, 2266.

21 Keohane P., Brown B., Grimble G. & Silk D.B.A. (1982) Effect of protein composition and hydrolysis procedures on intestinal handling of protein hydrolysates in man. *Clin. Sci.* **62**, 478.

22 Crane C.W. (1969) Some aspects of protein absorption and malabsorption. In *Malabsorption*, eds. R.H. Girdwood and A.N. Smith, p. 33. University Press, Edinburgh.

23 Fordtran J.S. & Locklear J.W. (1966) Ionic constituents and osmolality of gastric and small intestinal fluids after eating. *Am. J. Dig. Dis.* **11**, 503.

24 Ladas S., Isaacs P.E.T., Ureski Y., *et al* (1981) Are the jejunal luminal contents always iso-osmolar? *Gut* **22**, A868.

25 Sladen G.E. & Dawson A.M. (1969) Interrelationships between the absorptions of glucose, sodium and water by the normal human jejunum. *Clin. Sci.* **36**, 119.

26 Silk D.B.A., Fairclough P.D., Park N.J., Lane A.E., Webb J.P.W., Clark M.L. & Dawson A.M. (1975) A study of relations between the absorption of amino acids, dipeptides, water and electrolytes in the normal human jejunum. *Clin. Sci. Mol. Med.* **49**, 401.

27 Sladen G.E. & Dawson A.M. (1970) Effect of bicarbonate on sodium absorption by the human jejunum. *Nature* (London) **218**, 267.

28 Fordtran J.S., Rector F.C. Jr & Carter N.W. (1968) The mechanisms of sodium absorption in the human small intestine. *J. Clin. Invest.* **47**, 884.

29 Turnberg L.A., Fordtran J.S., Carter N.W. & Rector F.C. Jr (1970) Mechanism of bicarbonate absorption and its relationship to sodium transport in the human jejunum. *J. Clin. Invest.* **49**, 548.

30 Russell R.I. (1975) Elemental diets. *Gut* **16**, 68.

31 Koretz R.L. & Meyer J.H. (1980) Elemental diets—facts and fantasies. *Gastroenterology* **78**, 393.

32 Jones B.J.M., Lees R., Andrews J., *et al* (1980) Elemental and polymeric tube feeding in patients with normal gastrointestinal function: a controlled trial. *Gut* **21**, A905.

33 Jones D.C., Rich A.J., Wright P.D. & Johnston I.P.A. (1980) Comparison of proprietary elemental and whole-protein diets in unconscious patients with head injury. *Br. Med. J.* **1**, 1493.

34 Casewell M.W. (1979) Nasogastric feeds as a source of Klebsiella infection for intensive care patients. *Res. Clin. Forums* **1**, 101.

35 Bastow M.D., Allison S.P. & Greaves P. (1981) Study of microbial contamination of nasogastric feeds. In *Proceedings 3rd European Congress on Parenteral and Enteral Nutrition*, p 75.

36 Keighley M.R.B., Mogg B., Bentley S. & Allan C. (1982) 'Home brew' compared with commercial preparations for enteral feeding. *Br. Med. J.* **1**, 163.

37 Keohane P.P. & Silk D.B.A. (1983) Indications for use of mercury tipped nasogastric feeding tubes. *Clin. Nutr.* (in press).

38 Metz G., Dilawari J. & Kellock T.D. (1978) Simple technique for naso-enteric feeding. *Lancet* **ii**, 454.

39 Dobbie R.P. & Buttervich O.D. (1977) Continuous pump/tube enteric hyperalimentation—use in esophageal disease. *J. Parent. Ent. Nutr.* **1**, 100.

40 Atkinson M., Walford S. & Allison S.P. (1979) Endoscopic insertion of fine bore feeding tubes. *Lancet* **ii**, 829.

41 Keohane P.P., Attrill H. & Silk D.B.A. (1983) Endoscopic placement of fine bore nasogastric and nasoenteric feeding tubes. *Clin. Nutr.* **1**, 245.

42 Bunch G.A. & Shields R. (1969) Absorption of water and electrolytes by the human small intestine after surgical operations. *Br. J. Surg.* **52**, 708.

43 Harrower H.W. (1968) Postoperative ileus. *Am. J. Surg.* **110**, 369.

44 Sagar S., Harland P. & Shields R. (1979) Early postoperative feeding with elemental diet. *Br. Med. J.* **1**, 293.

45 Yeung C.K., Young G.A., Hackett A.F. & Hill G.L. (1978) Fine needle catheter jejunostomy—an assessment of a new method of nutritional support after major gastrointestinal surgery. *Br. J. Surg.* **66**, 727.

46 Jones B.J.M., Payne S. & Silk D.B.A. (1980) Indications for pump assisted enteral feeding. *Lancet* **i**, 1057.

47 Lee H.A. & Hartley T.F. (1975) A method of determining daily nitrogen requirements. *Postgrad. Med. J.* **51**, 441.

48 Kaminski M.V. (1976) Enteral hyperalimentation. *Surg. Gynae. Obstet.* **143**, 12.

49 Lee H.A. (1978) Parenteral nutrition. In *Nutrition in the Clinical Management of Disease*, eds. W.T. Dickerson and H.A. Lee, pp. 349–76. Edward Arnold, London.

50 Silk D.B.A. (1980) Enteral nutrition. *Hosp. Update* **8** 761.

51 McMichael H.B. (1979) Complications of enteral nutrition. *Res. Clin. For.* **1**, 107.

52 Tweedle D.E.F., Skidmore F.D., Gleave E.N., *et al* (1979) Nutritional support for patients undergoing surgery for cancer of the head and neck. *Res. Clin. For.* **1**, 59.

Chapter 8
Parenteral Feeding

Parenteral nutrition is indicated only when the nutritional requirements of the malnourished patient cannot be provided by the enteral route. There is a clearly identifiable group of post-operative patients with impaired gastrointestinal function who cannot be fed enterally, and require parenteral nutrition. In some patients, however, a trial of enteral feeding may be warranted and, if doubt exists, we have always been prepared to persevere with enteral feeding for a few days before resorting to parenteral nutrition. Adopting such a bias towards enteral feeding, we have found it necessary to resort to the use of parenteral feeding in only 25% of patients requiring nutritional support at Central Middlesex Hospital during the last three years. Although the mortality of our patients receiving parenteral nutrition is high (45% in our series of 84 patients), parenteral nutrition does provide a vital link in the chain of therapy for many patients, particularly those who have sustained severe injury.

Parenteral nutrition can be more hazardous than enteral nutrition. Table 8.1 highlights the major considerations of parenteral nutrition.

THE CATHETER

Since the outset of our nutrition programme, we have used silicone elastomer catheters. The reason for this choice is that these catheters have more favourable handling properties which are not lost during prolonged catheter placement, and they are less thrombogenic than polyvinyl, polyethylene or Teflon catheters [1]. We now routinely use a 35 cm long silicone feeding catheter (Vygon Nutricath S, code 2180.20) with a 25 cm long multipurpose extension tube (Vygon, code 220.02).

Catheter entry site

Infusion solutions for parenteral nutrition have high osmolalities and are sclerosant if given through short catheters into periph-

Table 8.1   Major considerations of parenteral nutrition.

Type of feeding catheter to be used
Choice of entry site for the infusion of nutrient solutions
Type of infusion system to be used
Nutrition regimen to be prescribed

eral veins. Similarly, infusion through long plastic catheters, threaded through antecubital veins terminating in the superior vena cava, is notorious for causing thrombophlebitis [2].

One of the safest methods of introducing these solutions is directly into the superior vena cava via subclavian vein catheterisation [3, 4]. In this way solutions with a concentration of 1500 mosmols can be infused through a short catheter at a rate of 2–3 ml/minute, while being diluted a thousand fold by a blood flow of 2–3 litres/minute. The entry site of the catheter is in a large vein, which decreases the likelihood of thrombophlebitis [5]. Our route of choice is the infraclavicular approach to the subclavian vein. The cutaneous entry site of the catheter is in the pectoral skin below the clavicle. This is an excellent place to keep clean and dress because it is flat, relatively immobile and does not collect perspiration and other secretions. Moreover, the patient's arm and neck remain free for normal motion.

In patients with clotting disorders, recent cervical surgery and severe obstructive airways disease, the subclavian approach should be avoided and the internal jugular route used [2], preferably with a skin tunnel (see later).

Catheter placement

Catheter placement should be performed by an experienced clinician, under aseptic conditions, preferably in an operating theatre [2, 6]. Parenteral nutrition is *never* an emergency procedure, and the complication rate of catheter placement is inversely proportional to the experience of the inserter [7] and is usually high in catheterisations done in an emergency [6].

Skin tunnelling

As the later text will show, one of the major complications of parenteral nutrition is catheter sepsis. Evidence points to the fact that this usually arises as a result of introduction of organisms via the catheter or the entry site itself [8]. When short catheters are used the infusion apparatus is attached close to the entry site. In contrast, if long catheters are used, the end point of the catheter can be tunnelled subcutaneously, so that junction between catheter and infusion apparatus is separated from the entry site. Using such a tunnelling technique [9], Powell-Tuck [10, 11] has reported a lower incidence of septicaemia compared to some of the other reported series [12, 13].

We have confirmed these observations, and in a prospective controlled clinical trial have observed a significantly lower incidence of catheter-related sepsis in the group of patients whose feeding catheter was tunnelled subcutaneously compared to those whose infusion apparatus was directly attached to the catheter close to the entry site [14].

Technique of catheter placement

There follows a description of the technique used at the Central Middlesex Hospital.

The patient is placed in the supine position, with 5° head-down tilt to avoid the risk of air embolus during vein puncture. The skin beneath the midpoint of the left clavicle is infiltrated with 1–2% lignocaine and a 1 cm skin incision is made. (It is helpful to identify the position of the subclavian vein using a long 20 gauge needle mounted on a syringe.) The needle is directed between the clavicle and the first rib, angled towards the tip of a finger held in the suprasternal notch. When blood is aspirated freely, the needle direction and depth are used as a guide to the insertion of a cannula through the skin incision into the subclavian vein. When free reflux of blood through the plastic sheath confirms the position, the silicone catheter is advanced 20–30 cm so that its tip lies in the distal part of the superior vena cava.

A skin tunnel is created under local anaesthesia by the use of an introducer inserted through a point about 10 cm below and medial to the incision and passed upwards to the incision. With the hub removed the proximal end of the catheter is passed backwards through the introducer so that it emerges into the anterior chest wall 10–15 cm below the clavicle. The infraclavicular entry incision is closed with fine nylon sutures, and the catheter is sutured to the chest wall close to its exit from the skin tunnel. In order to avoid unwanted tugging of the feeding catheter caused by movements of the infusion apparatus, the sterilised extension tube is attached to the feeding catheter and the infusion apparatus attached to this (Fig. 8.1).

Dressing

After insertion of the catheter, the entry site incision and the skin tunnel exit sites are sprayed with iodine and Opsite skin spray.

The skin tunnel exit site is then covered with a semipermeable adhesive dressing (Steripad 12.5 × 10 cm, Johnson & Johnson, Slough).

It has been traditional nursing practice to re-dress the catheter entry site every 48 hours and when necessary [15, 16]. We, as well as others [10], do not agree with this practice, and only take the dressings down if there are clinical suggestions or signs of catheter-related sepsis.

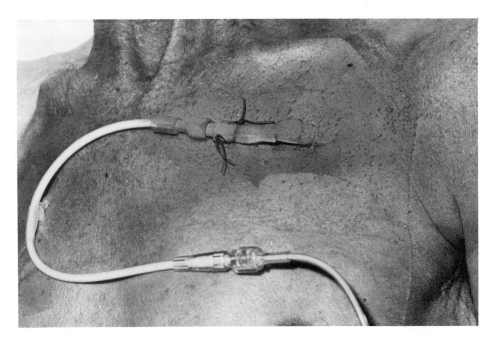

Fig. 8.1 Silicone feeding catheter in place. Note the separation of the infraclavicular entry incision from the site of exit of the feeding catheter from the subcutaneous skin tunnel. To avoid 'tugging' forces exerted by the infusion apparatus on the feeding catheter, the extension tube is connected to the feeding catheter and the infusion apparatus to this.

Checking the catheter position

After catheter insertion 5% dextrose should be infused. As soon as flow into the system is started, the bottle should be brought down to below the level of the heart, allowing backflow of blood into the infusion tubing, thereby confirming positioning of the catheter in the intravascular space. Hypertonic parenteral infusion should never be started until the position of the catheter has been checked radiographically (Fig. 8.2).

Complications of catheter insertion

The common complications are listed in Table 8.2, and involve the pleural space, intravascular space, mediastinum and nerve damage.

Central venous thrombosis

It is now generally accepted that the incidence of central venous thrombosis is less when silicone rather than plastic catheters are used [1, 17]. Although multiple factors have been implicated in

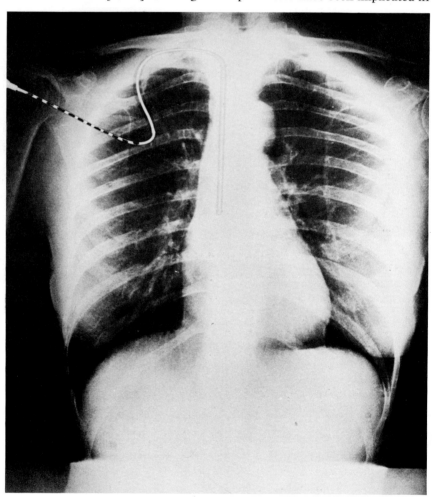

Fig. 8.2. Chest x-ray showing a silicone feeding catheter positioned via the right intraclavicular vein, the tip lying in the superior vena cava. For clarity of presentation the outline of the tube has been enhanced by a medical artist.

the initiation of central venous thrombosis (Table 8.3), the reason that silicone catheters are less thrombogenic is most likely due to the fact that they cause less endothelial damage than plastic catheters [18]. In the initial studies of central venous thrombosis, in which plastic catheters were largely used, an overall clinical frequency of 2.1% was reported [19]. Autopsy examinations of the central veins in patients who died while receiving parenteral nutrition via plastic catheters, though clearly dealing with a high risk group with a low flow state prior to death, showed a thrombosis incidence of as high as 27–71% [6, 19–21]. Prospective studies involving venography and the use of silicone catheters suggest an overall incidence of symptomatic and asymptomatic thrombosis of 4% [18], which substantiates the recommendations following the use of silicone catheters.

Table 8.2 Complications of catheter insertion.

Central vein thrombosis
Haemopericardium, hydropericardium and tamponade
Arrythmias (line on tricuspid valve)
Pneumothorax
Haemothorax
Hydrothorax (intrapleural infusion)
Air embolism
Tracheal puncture
Arterial puncture
Haematoma
Nerve injury—phrenic nerve, brachial plexus, recurrent laryngeal nerve

Table 8.3 Factors implicated in the initiation of central venous thrombosis.

Thrombus formation on the fibrin sheath surrounding the catheter
Endothelial damage caused by the tip of the catheter
Catheter infection
Misplacement in a small diameter tributary
Acid pH of infusion solutions
Hypertonicity of infusion solutions
Duration of parenteral nutrition

The main dangers of central vein thrombosis are the risk of pulmonary embolism [6], the development of the superior vena cava syndrome and septic thrombophlebitis, which has a high mortality rate [19, 22].

As there is some evidence that low-dose heparin infusion may prevent the formation of a fibrin sheath around the feeding catheter [23], we now routinely add 1000 units to our 3 litre delivery bag system. The incidence of thrombophlebitis is not altered by using millipore filters, so we do not advocate their use [24].

Once the clinical signs of central vein thrombosis develop, the feeding catheter should be removed, the patient heparinised, and then maintained on anticoagulants for six months.

Insertion of the relatively stiff plastic catheters into the right side of the heart may cause acute bacterial endocarditis, arrythmias or perforation of the atria and ventricles, resulting in fatal cardiac tamponade [25]. Fortunately, these complications are rare.

Pneumothorax

A clinically significant pneumothorax has occurred on at least two occasions at Central Middlesex during the last three years (Fig. 8.3). This, and the other complications involving the pleural space, such a haemothorax, hydrothorax and chylothorax (thoracic duct damage), are usually recognised clinically or by chest x-rays taken routinely to localise the position of the catheter. They should be treated by standard means. if the catheter is still in the bloodstream and the problem is under control, there may be no reason to remove the catheter.

Air embolism

This is an unusual but dramatic complication that is easily avoidable. It may occur in three ways:
1   During the process of catheter insertion when the syringe is removed to thread the catheter [26]. This can be prevented if the patient performs the Valsalva manoeuvre during catheter insertion. Application of moderate amounts of positive end expiratory pressure (PEEP) during catheterisation will prevent this complication in patients on a ventilator.
2   During tubing changes [27] which can be prevented as in 1.
3   After the catheter has been taken out and before the tract can seal [28]. To prevent this, white soft paraffin ointment and a small occlusive dressing should be placed over the insertion site for 24 hours.

Nerve injuries

These do occasionally occur, particularly to the brachial plexus. The catheter should be removed, the patient given physiotherapy and recovery is usually complete.

Catheter-related sepsis

The most frequent and potentially serious complication in patients receiving parenteral nutrition is catheter-related sepsis.

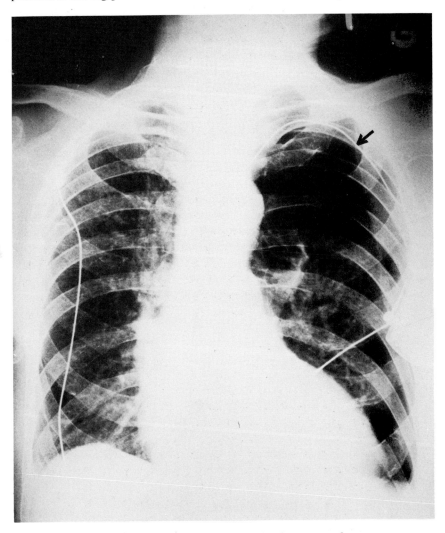

Fig. 8.3 Chest x-ray showing left pneumothorax that has occurred as a result of inserting a parenteral feeding catheter into the left subclavian vein (arrowed).

Of 37 series reviewed by Allen [29], the septicaemia rate varied from 0% to 93% [30, 31].

All the evidence points to the fact that septicaemia is most commonly related to growth of organisms along the side of the catheter within the percutaneous insertion site, or growth of organisms down the catheter due to breaks in a closed system [8, 29].

Table 8.4 lists the commonly isolated organisms from patients with catheter-related septicaemia.

There is no doubt that the incidence of septicaemia can be reduced with experience, and this can be embodied in the formation of a nutrition team [32] which should have primary responsibility for the care of all patients receiving parenteral nutrition (see Chapter 2).

At Central Middlesex Hospital over 20% of our patients developed a catheter-related septicaemia during the first 1000 patient days of parenteral nutrition [33]. Since the employment of a nursing sister with sole responsibilities for the nursing care of the catheter, improved nursing techniques, and increased experience of the physicians in the nutritional team, the incidence of catheter-related sepsis has been reduced to 4%.

Prevention of sepsis. The following rigorous protocols are adhered to in order to prevent catheter-related sepsis (Table 8.5):
1   The silicone catheters which are tunnelled subcutaneously are inserted by the same experienced operator under fully sterile conditions in theatres.

Table 8.4   Microbial pathogens causing catheter related septicaemia.

GRAM-POSITIVE COCCI
Staphylococcus aureus
Staphylococcus epidermidis
Streptococcal species, alpha or non-haemolytic
Enterococcus

GRAM-NEGATIVE BACTERIA
Klebsiella spp.
Pseudomonas spp.
Escherichia coli
Enterobacter spp.
Proteus rettgeri
ANAEROBIC BACTERIA
Bacteroides spp.

FUNGI
Candida spp.
Torulopsis spp.

Table 8.5 Prevention of catheter-related sepsis.

Establish a nutrition team

Separate infraclavicular catheter entry site
from exit site on anterior chest wall by
subcutaneous tunnelling

Nursing care of catheter entry sites
responsibility of nutrition nurse

Dress catheter entry site only when
clinically indicated*

In-line millipore filters not used*

No topical antibiotic ointments or sprays
used

Low dose heparin infused with nutrients

Change infusion apparatus under aseptic
conditions every 24 hours

Use of feeding lines restricted to nutrient
solutions only

* Local practice and somewhat controversial

2   The nursing of the catheter entry site is the responsibility of
the nutrition nurse. Once sited and dressed (see p. 104, 105)
neither the infraclavicular catheter entry site nor the skin tunnel
exit sites are tampered with unless clinically indicated. Various
recommendations have been made as to how frequently the
catheter entry and exit sites should be dressed, ranging from
every 48 hours [16] to once a week [34], and we feel that our
improved figures justify the more conservative approach. At
present we are using a semi-permeable membrane type of
dressing. Although it has been recently suggested that the use of
such dressings may be associated with a higher incidence of
catheter-related sepsis than standard gauze/tape dressings [35],
we again feel that our improved figures justify their use.
3   We do not use in-line millipore filters [24], nor do we use
topical antibiotic ointments or sprays, as there is evidence that
their use causes the frequency of colonisation of the catheter
entry site with Candida to increase [36]. Small doses of heparin
are infused (1000 U/3 litres) in the hopes of reducing the
incidence of septicaemia [23].
4   The infusion apparatus should be changed daily using an
aseptic technique, with the nurse and patient wearing a mask,
and the nurse a gown and gloves. Although the recommendation

of changing the infusion apparatus every 24 hours is based on carefully performed studies [37], there is some evidence that using administration sets for 48 hours does not increase the incidence of catheter-related sepsis [38].

5   The administration of blood products, antibiotics and other medications through the feeding catheter is banned. *There should be no exceptions.* Nutritional additives such as vitamins, trace elements and haematinics should all be added to the infusion solutions by the pharmacist under sterile conditions before they are delivered to the wards.

Diagnosis of catheter-related sepsis. Patients receiving parenteral nutrition frequently have infections at other sites [5], and problems in diagnosis always arise when signs of sepsis, such as chills, fever and leucocytosis develop. Up to two-thirds of positive blood cultures may turn out to have originated from sites other than the catheter tip [39]. Clues to the origin of the septicaemia are that positive cultures of Staphylococcus or Candida are most likely to be of catheter origin, whereas up to 80% of septicaemias not related to the catheter are likely to be due to Gram-negative organisms [39]. In practical terms, we recommend the following course of action if catheter-related sepsis is suspected:

1   Clinical examination.
2   Full blood picture.
3   Swabs from the catheter entry site and skin tunnel exit sites.
4   Peripheral venous blood cultures.
5   Cultures of sputum and urine.
6   Appropriate radiographs.

If there is another obvious source of sepsis (wound infection, pneumonia, urinary tract infection, intra-abdominal abscess), treat these first and continue parenteral nutrition. If no other source of infection becomes obvious and the fever continues for 24 hours, remove the catheter. Any patient with recurrent positive blood cultures should have the catheter removed. When the catheter is removed, the tip should be cut off into a sterile tube and smeared on appropriate culture media for both bacteria and fungi.

Treatment

Both the diagnosis and treatment of catheter-related sepsis depend upon removal of the feeding catheter and we do not believe in routine initial treatment. If tissue invasion with fungus has occurred [40] or if other septic bacterial foci are identified, treatment with catheter removal alone is not adequate, and appropriate antibiotics or antifungal agents in adequate dosages for systemic therapy should be given.

Careful observation of the patient is essential following removal of a catheter causing sepsis. If the clinical picture is compatible with persistent or serious infection or if blood cultures remain positive, appropriate antibiotics or antifungal treatment should be instituted [29].

If a catheter needs to be removed, we usually maintain the patient on 5% dextrose solutions administered via a peripheral line for 24 hours in order to allow the bacteraemia to clear. In practice the fever usually clears by the time 24–48 hours of peripheral feeding has elapsed and the cultures of the catheter tip and blood have been returned. At this stage, a new feeding catheter can be positioned and parenteral nutrition recommenced. If a persistent bacteraemia persists, it is probably better to complete the course of antibiotic therapy before recommencing parenteral nutrition.

THE NUTRITION REGIME

Principles of a nutrition regime

Parenteral nutrition implies the intravenous administration of sufficient nitrogen to provide essential and non-essential amino acids for protein synthesis, calories to meet energy requirements and both to minimise or reverse peripheral protein breakdown. In addition, the electrolyte, vitamin, trace element and haematinic requirements of the patient must be met. One of the basic principles of the nutrition regime is that the nitrogen and energy sources should be infused simultaneously [41], in order to maximise the rate of protein synthesis.

Nitrogen source

Although early clinical experiences suggested that the possibly less well-defined partial enzymic hydrolysates of whole protein exerted as good an effect on nitrogen balance as the more exactly defined synthetic L-amino acid solutions [42–44], their use has been superseded by the pure L-amino acid solutions. Some, but not all, of the more widely used L-amino acid formulations are listed in Table 8.6.

It is generally agreed that the essential amino acids should comprise 40% or so of the total amino acid content by weight. There is considerable controversy, however, as to whether glycine, present in comparatively large proportions in some of these solutions (e.g. Aminoplex 12 and 14), acts as an efficient

Table 8.6 Some parenteral amino acid solutions used in the UK and USA.

	Nitrogen (g/litre)	Sodium (mmol/litre)	Potassium (mmol/litre)	Magnesium (mmol/litre)	Calcium (mmol/litre)	Phosphate (mmol/litre)	Chloride (mmol/litre)	Acetate (mmol/litre)	Comments
Vamin N* (Kabivitrum)	9.4	50	20	1.5	2.5	—	55	—	Available with glucose and fructose
Aminoplex 12	12.4	35	30	2.5	—	—	67	—	Extra gram of nitrogen in Aminoplex 14 is all glycine
Aminoplex 14 (Geistlich)	13.4	35	30	—	—	—	79	—	
Synthamin 9	9.3	73	60	5	—	30	70	100	Electrolyte free versions available
Synthamin 14	14.4	73	60	5	—	30	70	130	
Synthamin 17 (Travenol)	16.9	73	60	5	—	30	70	150	
Aminofusin L Forte (BDH Pharmaceuticals)	15.2	40	30	5	—	—	27	—	Low essential amino acid composition
FreAmine II (Boots)	12.6	10	—	—	—	10	—	—	

* High nitrogen version available in Sweden

precursor for synthesis of other amino acids or is effectively utilised as an energy source via gluconeogenesis.

It is interesting that those who claim that some of the amino acid solutions are formulated with inappropriately large amounts of glycine [45] base their assertions, at least in part, on results of studies where oral loading techniques were used [46]. Although there is evidence that 6–8% of infused glycine is lost in the urine during the first three days [47], we have yet to be convinced one way or the other and would at present still recommend the routine use of any of these amino acid formulations. We are, however, currently investigating the problem by performing protein turnover studies using a ^{13}C-leucine labelling technique in patients randomised to receive crossover infusions of crystalline amino acid formulations containing relatively high or low glycine contents.

For simplicity, clinicians are advised to work with a small number of stock solutions, not the least of all because it facilitates purchasing by the Pharmacy Department. The author has a personal preference for the Synthamin range of solutions, for although there are three solutions (9.3, 14,4, 16.9 g N/l) the proportions of individual amino acids in each solution is fixed. The three solutions, Synthamin 9, 14 and 17 can therefore be used respectively to treat patients with low, intermediate and high nitrogen requirements. In practice few of our patients requiring parenteral nutrition have nitrogen requirements as low as 9.3 g/day, so the bulk of our patients receive Synthamin 14 or 17.

The energy source

In considering energy sources in parenteral nutrition, two important questions have arisen. The first surrounds the use of glucose or alternative carbohydrate energy sources and the second concerns the question of whether carbohydrate should be used as the sole source of energy or whether it should be combined with fat.

Glucose

Glucose is the predominant form in which orally ingested carbohydrate reaches the peripheral organs in man, so it would seem logical that it should be the carbohydrate energy source of choice in parenteral nutrition regimes, particularly since it is metabolised by peripheral tissue as well as in the liver. With the exception of red blood cells and brain tissue, cellular glucose uptake is insulin-dependent. Some severely stressed patients are unable to mobilise and utilise insulin normally [48], and this so-called insulin resistance has been used as an argument against the use of glucose in such patients [49], and has prompted the search for alternative carbohydrate energy sources. In our experience, however, careful administration of insulin supplements circumvents this problem and, as the ensuing text will show, none of the alternative carbohydrate energy sources so far proposed are without problems or side-effects (Table 8.7).

The strongest arguments that can be cited in favour of glucose as the carbohydrate energy source of choice relate to the existence of two important mechanisms that regulate its breakdown, thereby ensuring controlled energy production. Thus, although a number of biochemical reactions are involved in the conversion of glucose to energy (Fig. 8.4), overall energy production is regulated by the action of two enzymes involved in the early steps of glucose metabolism. The first, glucokinase, is responsible for converting glucose to glucose-6-phosphate; this enzyme has a low substrate specificity, which means that glucose-6-phosphate is most rapidly produced when the concentrations of glucose are high, usually above circulating blood levels. The second, phosphofructokinase, is responsible for catalysing the hydrolysis of fructose-6-phosphate to fructose-1,6-diphosphate and is the most important of the two regulatory

Table 8.7 Carbohydrate energy sources in parenteral nutrition.

Carbohydrate energy source	Problems
Glucose	Hyperglycaemia
Fructose Sorbitol	Uncontrolled metabolism Reduction in hepatic protein synthesis rates Lactic acidosis
Xylitol	Uncontrolled metabolism Triglyceridaemia Oxalaemia, oxaluria Hyperuricaemia
Ethanol	Toxic effects on liver, pancreas, bone marrow, central and peripheral nervous systems
Maltose Glucose oligosaccharides	Metabolism limited and renal losses high

enzymes. Its activity is dependent upon intracellular concentrations of ATP, ADP and citrate. Thus, in the presence of low concentrations of ATP and citrate and high concentrations of ADP, glucose breakdown is stimulated, and vice versa.

At Central Middlesex Hospital, we routinely use glucose as our carbohydrate energy source in parenteral nutrition and administer insulin if and when necessary.

Sorbitol and fructose metabolism (Fig. 8.4)

Unlike glucose, sorbitol and fructose are both metabolised mostly in the liver [50, 51]. Sorbitol is oxidised to fructose by sorbitol

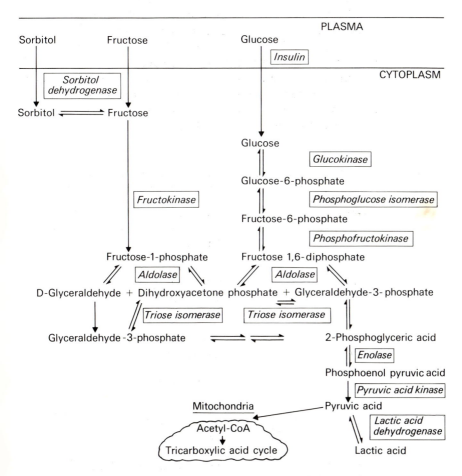

Fig. 8.4 Pathways of sorbitol, fructose and glucose metabolism in the liver.

dehydrogenase and, thereafter, its metabolism is the same as that of fructose.

Fructose has been advocated as having advantages over glucose as a carbohydrate energy source in parenteral nutrition, largely because its cellular uptake is non-insulin-dependent [52] and because it is more rapidly metabolised than glucose [53, 54]. The first step in fructose metabolism is its phosphorylation by fructokinase. Since the controlling enzymes in the glycolytic pathway can exert no limitation on the rate of hepatic fructose metabolism, there is no limit to the amount of fructose converted to fructose-1-phosphate by frucktokinase [55–57]. Furthermore, it should be remembered that unlike glucokinase, fructokinase has a high substrate affinity. The consequence of these above events is that triose production (dihydroxyacetone phosphate and glyceraldehyde), and therefore energy production, is uncontrolled. Although this alone can be viewed as a disadvantage in parenteral nutrition, there is additional experimental evidence to show that the rapid accumulation of fructose-1-phosphate leads to depletion of ATP and sequestration of inorganic phosphate [56] which in turn results in a reduction in the rate of hepatic protein synthesis [58].

As mentioned above, hepatic uptake of fructose is twice that of glucose [59, 60]. Even in the normal situation, reverse glycolysis in the liver results in the conversion of only 70% of an administered dose to glucose [56]. Under anaerobic conditions, however, fructose metabolism is increased and the only end product is lactate [61]. Patients requiring parenteral nutrition often have high lactate levels even before treatment [62], so that on commencement lactate production will be appreciable. Overall, then, the rate of utilisation of fructose and sorbitol will depend upon metabolism of lactate [62], and not the rate of substrate clearance from blood. The occurrence of lactic acidosis during parenteral nutrition with fructose and sorbitol has now indeed been well documented [63] so these sugars cannot be recommended in preference to glucose.

Xylitol metabolism

Xylitol is a five-carbon alcohol, which, as in the case of sorbitol, is oxidised in the liver [64]; oxidation by polyol dehydrogenase is the initial step in its metabolism. What has been said for sorbitol and fructose is true for xylitol, namely that a load of xylitol has to be taken care of entirely by the liver, and there is no limitation to the amount metabolised by controlling enzymes in the glycolytic pathway. Although appreciable (60–75%) amounts of xylitol are eventually converted to glucose [65], because of the lack of control of its metabolic rate accumulation of high concentrations of intermediate and end products of metabolism can occur. The use of xylitol in parenteral nutrition has thus been associated with triglyceridaemia, oxalaemia, oxaluria and hyperuricaemia [66]. In addition to these problems, up to 20% of administered xylitol may be lost in the urine [49, 67] due to the fact that pentitols are not reabsorbed in kidney tubules [68]. Xylitol, like sorbitol and fructose cannot, therefore, be recommended as an alternative to glucose as the carbohydrate energy source in parenteral nutrition.

Ethanol

In the view of the author, the use of ethanol as an energy source in parenteral nutrition is completely prohibited on account of the toxic effects it exerts on the liver, pancreas, heart, bone marrow and central, as well as peripheral, nervous systems.

Maltose

The disaccharide maltose provides double the calories compared to iso-osmotic solutions of glucose, and thus represents a theoretical alternative to glucose as an energy source and, by virtue of the fact that on a calorie to calorie comparison maltose exerts a lower osmolality than glucose, it could be administered via a peripheral, rather than central, vein.

The use of maltose would appear, however, to have major drawbacks, particularly in respect of renal losses, which may be as high as 50% of dose administered [69–71]. The reason for this is likely to be that a major site of hydrolysis is the proximal renal tubule, and that like the gut hydrolysis proceeds faster than glucose reabsorption from the proximal tubule. In turn this leads to high renal losses of glucose despite normal blood glucose levels [70, 71]. We believe that it will be unlikely that maltose will ever find wide-scale clinical usage as a carbohydrate energy source in parenteral nutrition.

Glucose oligosaccharides

An extension of the work with maltose has been to investigate the possible usefulness of glucose oligosaccharide mixtures as hypotonic carbohydrate energy sources in parenteral nutrition. The first to be studied was the $\alpha 1$–4, $\alpha 1$–6 linked glucose oligosaccharide, Caloreen. As with maltose, however, renal losses were high, up to 45%, making it unsuitable for further clinical use [72]. Further studies have now been performed with a more highly purified α1–4 linked glucose oligosaccharide containing a predominance of 2–8 glucose units [73]. Again, significant urinary losses occurred, particularly at high infusion rates, and up to 40% of the excreted sugar was found to be in the form of higher oligosaccharide chains. These findings, therefore, suggest that the ability of man to metabolise infused glucose oligosaccharides is limited, and that in the future they will not turn out to be a satisfactory alternative to glucose as the major carbohydrate energy source in parenteral nutrition.

Fat emulsions in parenteral nutrition

The use of fat emulsions in parenteral nutrition has a number of advantages [74]:
1   Fat is a concentrated source of energy; it provides 9 kcal per gram, and can thus furnish a greater number of calories in a smaller volume than carbohydrate energy sources.
2   Even when an adequate carbohydrate energy source is used, the use of fat as a calorie source is important, for it prevents essential fatty acid deficiency.
3   Even a 20% fat emulsion is not considered hypertonic.
4   The infusion of fat emulsion does not cause a diuresis, and there is no loss of the infused fat emulsion in the urine or faeces.
5   Fat can function as a carrier of the fat-soluble vitamins in the form of fatty acid esters.

Fat emulsion preparations

There are a number of fat emulsions available for clinical use. The basic ingredients of these solutions are similar in that they contain a vegetable oil, an emulsifier and a polyhydric alcohol to render the solution isotonic. Experiences of fat emulsions in this country are largely restricted to Intralipid (10 and 20%) which contains soya bean vegetable oil, egg yolk phosphatide as the emulsifier and the polyol glycerol.

Utilisation and metabolism of fat emulsions (Fig. 8.5)

The rate of elimination of infused Intralipid from blood is high, ranging from 3.8 in subjects fasting overnight and increasing to 10.9 g fat/kg body wt/24 hours in the post-operative period, after two days fasting [75, 76].

Triglycerides in fat emulsions are taken up by peripheral tissues and utilised in the same way as chylomicrons [77, 78]. Thus a requirement for uptake is prior lipolysis in the intravascular compartment by lipoprotein lipase [74]. Available evidence

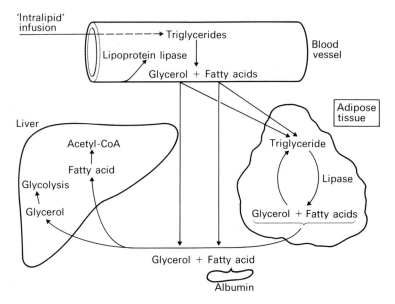

Fig. 8.5 Utilisation and metabolism of fat emulsions used in parenteral nutrition.

indicates that the fat emulsion Intralipid is hydrolysed by lipoprotein lipase at the same rate as chylomicrons [76, 79].

Energy is derived from both the glycerol and fatty acid moieties of the triglycerides contained in the fat emulsions. Glycerol enters the metabolic pathway of glucose breakdown via formation of L-glycerol-3-phosphate and dihydroxyacetone phosphate (3-carbon containing compounds shown in Fig. 8.4).

Fatty acid oxidation is accomplished by a sequence of reactions whereby one molecule of acetyl-CoA is generated and the fatty acyl chain shortened by a unit of 2 carbon atoms. Energy accrues on two accounts: first, because the production of acetyl-CoA in itself results in the formation of ATP; second, due to the fact that acetyl-CoA enters the tricarboxylic acid cycle yielding an additional 12 mols of ATP per mol of acetyl CoA oxidised.

The administration of fat emulsions will result in the production of energy in all situations where endogenous fat stores are normally being mobilised as part of the metabolic response to injury or starvation. The net effect of providing this energy source is similar to the net effect of endogeneous fat mobilisation, namely to prevent the breakdown of protein stores for energy production. The term 'nitrogen sparing effect' has been coined to describe this, and there has been, and will continue to be, a discussion about the optimal proportion of fat to carbohydrate that will result in the maximum nitrogen sparing effect in different conditions.

Fat or carbohydrate?

Early comparisons of the nitrogen-sparing effect of intravenous fat and glucose in moderately hypermetabolic patients showed few differences [80–84]. However, in the most recently performed study, Hill and colleagues [85] have shown quite clearly that the weight gain noted when glucose alone was used as the energy source in surgical gastroenterological patients, was due to gains in total body water and not protein. Only when a mixture of fat and glucose was used were significant gains in total body protein noted.

We have taken note of this study and now routinely use an energy source based on glucose and fat in our parenteral nutrition regimes.

One important point does have to be made, however, and that is that the above studies [80–85] were performed, by and large, in moderately hypermetabolic patients. The final conclusion drawn, that a mixture of fat and glucose should be used as the non-protein energy in parenteral nutrition, may not necessarily apply to severely stressed hypermetabolic patients.

In some such patients there may be a lack of stimulation of endogenous lipid metabolism [86–88]. The cause is likely to be related to associated hormonal changes, in that response to severe injury in some patients is characterised by low blood levels of free fatty acids and ketones and high levels of glucose lactate and insulin [88]. Insulin, it will be remembered, exerts an antilipolytic effect [89]. There are thus grounds for believing that in these patients the use of fat emulsions would not have the expected nitrogen sparing effect and, indeed, there are now clinical studies in critically ill patients showing that the nitrogen sparing effect of fat emulsions is related to utilisation of glycerol and not to fatty acid content of the fat emulsions used [90, 91].

In other hypermetabolic patients, despite their ability to mobilise fat stores in response to stress, anaerobic metabolism may predominate [86] with concomitant production of lactate and conversion of acetyl-CoA to ketone bodies (acetoacetate, β-hydroxybutyrate and acetone) rather than entry into the tricarboxylic acid cycle. High blood ketones stimulate insulin secretion [66] with concomitant inhibition of lipolysis. This is the stage at which the patient is said to be fully 'keto-adapted' and, this being the case, there would be additional reasons for believing that glucose rather than a mixture of glucose and fat should be used as the non-protein energy source.

Until recently we had been swayed by the above discussion and by clinical data showing a more favourable effect on nitrogen balance in hypermetabolic patients when non-protein energy is administered in the form of glucose alone, compared with a combination of fat and glucose [92, 93]. Consequently, it had been our practice to routinely recommend the use of glucose alone as the energy source in all hypermetabolic patients with nitrogen requirements in excess of 18 g/day [2]. The exception to this was the recommendation that 1 litre of 20% Intralipid should be infused once a week to prevent the development of essential fatty acid deficiency.

Our whole thinking has been changed, however, since the publication by Kinney and colleagues of a study showing a significant utilisation of fat for energy in a group of 14 hypermetabolic patients [94] Although this work clearly needs confirming, we now use a mixture of glucose and fat as the non-protein energy source in all our patients receiving parenteral nutrition.

Essential fatty acid deficiency

The clinical characteristics of essential fatty acids (EFA) deficiency were first described in rats fed a fat-free diet by Burr and Burr [95]. The prominent features were a scaly skin, hair loss and skin sores. Similar lesions have now been reported in paediatric and adult patients treated with fat-free parenteral nutritional regimes.

The only fatty acid essential to man is linoleic acid (18:2 (Δ9, 12)). This acid is normally elongated and desaturated to form arachidonic acid (20:4 (Δ5, 8, 11, 14)). In the absence of linoleic acid, increased amounts of stearic acid (18:0) synthesised from non-fat precursors, is converted to oleic acid (18:1 (Δ9)) which in turn is converted to eicosatrienoic acid (20:3 (Δ5, 8, 11)). Consequently, on a fat free diet eicosatrienoic acid (triene) becomes detectable in plasma as levels of linoleic and arachidonic acids (tetraene) falls. This biochemical phenomenon led Holman [96] to define essential fatty acid deficiency by means of a triene:tetraene (20:3/20:4) ratio. A ratio of greater than 0.4 is taken as evidence of EFA deficiency. A recent clinical study has shown that all patients treated with a fat-free parenteral nutrition regime for 4 weeks have a ratio of greater than 0.4 [97].

The precise daily requirement of essential fatty acids in man is not known, although it has been estimated at 1–4% of the total caloric intake [97]. Estimation of plasma levels of arachiodonic and eicosatrienoic acids remains a research procedure requiring thin layer and gas liquid chromatography. In the day-to-day clinical setting, biochemical and clinical EFA deficiency can be prevented by infusing the equivalent of 1 litre of 20% Intralipid per week.

Calorie to nitrogen ratios in parenteral nutrition

The subject of non-protein energy to nitrogen ratios has been discussed in Chapter 6. In brief, it was concluded that the highest ratio (250:1) was most appropriate in those patients with low energy and nitrogen requirements, and that the lowest ratios (135:1) were most suited to the hypermetabolic patients with high energy and nitrogen requirements.

Various recommendations have been made for parenteral nutrition regimes. We have tended to use the 150:1 ratio recommended originally by Dudrick and Ruberg [98] and later by Peters and Fischer [99]. On face value, two recent studies [100, 101] suggest that this ratio is too high, and that a nitrogen intake in excess of 0.30 g N/kg per day is required to prevent net loss of body protein, which would result in the lowering of the ratio to 135:1.

It is a pity [102] that no attempts were made to assess the resting metabolic expenditure of the patients included in the above studies. Thus we can never be sure if the patients were in the anabolic phase of the metabolic response to injury, in which case positive nitrogen balance would be achieved with ease, or whether the patients were hypermetabolic and in the flow phase, in which case positive nitrogen balance would be virtually impossible to achieve in a milieu of elevated catecholamines and stress hormones.

In practice most clinicians will not be able to assess the resting metabolic expenditure of their patients, and the energy and nitrogen requirements are most simply assessed from measurements of using urea excretion (p. 59). Requirements are best calculated to exceed losses by 5 g nitrogen per day with a middle-of-the-road non-protein energy to nitrogen ratio of 150:1.

Electrolytes and trace elements

Close monitoring of electrolyte status is required, particularly in hypermetabolic patients, to avoid deficiency or excess. Tables 8.6 and 8.8 show how few preparations contain adequate amounts of electrolytes and trace elements. Although supplementary trace elements are probably not necessary for periods of less than 1 week, unless nutritional depletion has occurred prior to starting parenteral nutrition we routinely add 10 ml of Addamel (Table 8.8) to each 3 litre container of parenteral fluids.

Table 8.8 Recommended daily electrolyte and trace element requirements and available preparations*. Modified from [45] and [103].

	Na⁺ (mmol)	K⁺ (mmol)	Mg²⁺ (mmol)	Ca²⁺ (mmol)	Zn²⁺ (μmol)	Mn²⁺ (μmol)	Fe³⁺ (μmol)	Cu²⁺ (μmol)	Cl⁻ (mmol)	PO₄³⁻ (mmol)	F⁻ (μmol)	I⁻ (μmol)
Recommended daily requirement	70–220	60–120	5–20	5–10	50	7	70	5	70–220	20–40	50	1
Addamel (Kabivitrum) per 10 ml ampoule	—	—	1.5	5	20	40	50	5	13	—	50	1
Electrolyte A† (Travenol) per 500 ml	—	—	14	13	40	20	—	—	54	—	—	—
Electrolyte B† (Travenol) per 500 ml	—	30	—	—	—	—	—	—	—	30	—	—
Glucoplex 1600‡ (Geistlich) per 500 ml	25	15	1.25	—	23	—	—	—	33.5	9	—	—
Glucoplex 1000§ (Geistlich) per 500 ml	25	15	1.25	—	23	—	—	—	33.5	9	—	—

* Selenium and chromium not supplied by these products;
† Dextrose 20%; ‡ Dextrose 40%; § Dextrose 25%.

Vitamin sources (Table 8.9)

In the UK Solivito is the most complete source of water-soluble vitamins. However it contains insufficient B vitamins or vitamin C for hypermetabolic patients and such patients should receive 2 vials of Solivito per day plus 500 mg ascorbic acid daily. At the Central Middlesex Hospital, Solivito, Multibionta and Parentrovite are rotated on a daily basis.

Whenever possible alcoholics should be given thiamine (200 mg tds) orally to prevent development of the Wernicke–Korsakoff syndrome.

Vitlipid, a source of fat-soluble vitamins, should be added to Intralipid prior to administration. Both Vitlipid and Multibionta may contain too much vitamin A.

B vitamins are adversely affected by sunlight and infusions should be shielded by an opaque plastic bag.

THE DELIVERY SYSTEMS

One of the most important practical advances in parenteral nutrition during the last few years has been the development of a delivery system in which the daily requirements of parenteral fluids are mixed together and administered from a single 3 litre bag container [10, 104].

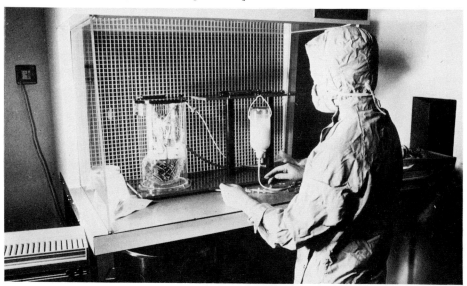

Fig. 8.6 Preparation of parenteral nutrition solutions in the pharmacy. Note the use of the laminar flow hood and the outer garments and hair covering caps worn by the pharmacist during the procedure.

Table 8.9 Vitamin solutions for intravenous infusion (modified from [45]).

| | Recommended daily intake | Parentrovite IVHP | | | | Vitlipid Adult | Intralipid 20% (500 ml) |
		Multibionta	Ampoules 1	Ampoules 2	Solivito		
B1 Thiamine (mg)	1.4	50	250	—	1.2	—	—
B2 Riboflavin (mg)	2.1	7.29	4.0	—	1.8	—	—
B6 Pyridoxine (mg)	2.1	15	50	—	2.0	—	—
B12 Cyanocobalamin (µg)	2.0	—	—	—	2.0	—	—
Nicotinamide (mg)	14	100	—	160	10	—	—
Biotin (mg)	0.35	—	—	—	0.3	—	—
Pantothenic acid/ dexpanthenol (mg)	14	25	—	—	10	—	—
Folic acid (mg)	2	—	—	—	0.2	—	—
C Ascorbic acid (mg)	35	500	—	500	30	—	—
D Calciferol (IU)	100	—	—	—	—	120	—
K Phytylmenaquinone (µg)	140	—	—	—	—	150	—
A Retinol (IU)	700	10000	—	—	—	2500	—
E Tocopheryl acetate (IU)	30	5	—	—	—	—	30

Modified from [45]

Preparation of fluids

All the patient's requirements of energy, amino acids, minerals, vitamins and trace elements are introduced into the 3 litre bag (B7992 3 l empty parenteral nutrition container, Travenol), using a scrupulous aseptic technique under a laminar flow hood with filtered air (Fig. 8.6).

Recommendations have been made that fat emulsions should not be mixed with other nutrients in the bag [105]. However, for a number of years an Intralipid-based feeding mixture has been successfully used in France [106, 107], and on the basis of this we have been routinely mixing 20% Intralipid with other nutrients in our 3 litre bag delivery system.

Over 50 patients at Central Middlesex Hospital have received this Intralipid-based feeding mixture and no untoward clinical side-effects have been noted. Although we have not specifically performed stability studies in our own mixtures, others have confirmed that minimal chemical and physical changes occur, providing standard aseptic mixing practices are followed [108].

The main advantage of the 3 litre bag delivery system is that the fluid can be delivered from the container through a single lead giving set and only one change is needed during each 24 hour period of infusion. We use the Travenol C 2071 sterile administration set.

The fluid can be allowed to flow under gravity but the use of a pump ensures a constant flow-rate and built in alarm systems remove the need for continuous attention. We use an Imed 922 volumetric infusion pump, and have found it reliable and capable of supplying fluids accurately over a wide range of infusion rates. If the outflow becomes obstructed, pressures sufficient to burst the catheter or disconnect the giving set do not build up. At the same time the pressure does not cut out altogether, so allowing blood to flow back into the catheter and, most important of all, the pump is designed in such a way that it is incapable of infusing air. Our complete parenteral nutrition delivery system is shown in Fig. 8.7.

The basic regimes

The two basic regimes for the 3 litre bag delivery system used at Central Middlesex Hospital (Table 8.10) are based on the use of Synthamin 14 and Synthamin 17 as the nitrogen source, and a mixture of dextrose and Intralipid as the energy source. Regime A (14.3 g N) has a non-protein energy to nitrogen ration (kcal/g N) of 196:1 and regime B (16.9 g N) has a corresponding ratio of 166:1.

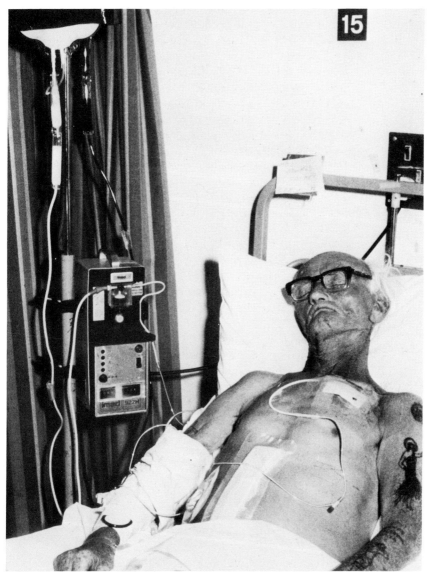

Fig. 8.7 Parenteral nutrition delivery system used routinely at Central Middlesex Hospital. Parenteral fluids, including 20% Intralipid are mixed together in the 3l bag (Travenol B7992 3l empty parenteral nutrition container) and delivered via the single lead giving set (Travenol C2071 sterile administration set) by means of an Imed 922 volumetric infusion pump.

Additives

The fat-soluble vitamin requirements are satisfied by adding 1 vial Vitlipid (Table 8.9) to the bag. We satisfy the water-soluble vitamin requirements by adding 1 vial Solivito, 1 vial Multibionta and ampoules 1 and 2 of Parentrovite IVHP in rotation on a daily basis. Hypermetabolic patients receive 2 vials of Solivito/day plus 500 mg ascorbic acid daily. B vitamins are adversely affected by sunlight, so the 3l dag should be covered by an opaque plastic bag.

Electrolytes A and B, it will be remembered (Table 8.8), are 20% dextrose solutions that contain mineral and trace elements (A) and phosphate (B). 1 vial Addamel is added in the hopes of satisfying additional trace element requirements.

If hyperglycaemia develops during parenteral nutrition soluble

Table 8.10 Breakdown of parenteral nutrition regimes A and B (units are mmol unless otherwise stated).

	VN*	E*	N*	Ratio	Na	K	Cl	PO_4	Ca	Mg	Zn	Mn
Regime A												
Synthamin	1000		14		73	60	70	30		5		
Intralipid 20%	500	1000						7.5				
Electrolyte A	500	400					54		13	14	0.04	0.02
Electrolyte B	500	400				30		30				
Dextrose 20%	500	400										
Total	3000	2200	14	159:1	73	90	124	67.5	13	19	0.04	0.02
Regime B												
Synthamin	1000		14		73	60	70	30		5		
Intralipid 20%	500	1000						7.5				
Electrolyte A	500	400					54		13	14	0.04	0.02
Electrolyte B	500	400				30		30				
Dextrose 20%	500	400										
Total	3000	2200	14	129:1	73	90	124	67.5	13	19	0.04	0.02

* VN = volume (ml); E = energy (Kcal); N = nitrogen (g); Ratio = non-protein energy to nitrogen ratio (kcal/g N).

insulin can be added, and we usually add 1000 units of heparin to the bag in the hopes of reducing the incidence of catheter-related sepsis [23].

Prescription for the regime (Fig. 8.8)

If it has been traditional for parenteral nutrition regimes to be prescribed on drug or standard intravenous therapy charts, the clinician is advised to change this. We have developed a 3 litre

CENTRAL MIDDLESEX HOSPITAL NUTRITIONAL SUPPORT SERVICE

3 LITRE BAG PARENTERAL NUTRITION PRESCRIPTION FORM

Name	Age	Hospital No.	Ward	Start Date	Completion Date

Diagnosis						
Basic Solutions	Volume	non N_2 Energy	N_2 g	Na^+ mmol	K^+ mmol	Batch No.
Synthamin 9 + electrolytes						
Synthamin 14 + electrolytes						
Synthamin 17 + electrolytes						
Synthamin 9 – electrolyte free						
Synthamin 14 – electrolyte free						
Synthamin 17 – electrolyte free						
Dextrose 50% (2000 kcal/l)						
Dextrose 20% (800 kcal/l)						
Electrolyte A (dextrose 20%)						
Electrolyte B (dextrose 20%)						
Dextrose 10% (400 kcal/l)						
5% Saline (855 kcal/l)						
1.8% (2N)Saline(300 kcal/l)						
0.9% (N) Saline(150 kcal/l)						
TOTALS						

Additives	Dose	Batch No.	
Potassium Chloride Inj. B.P. (20 mmol/10 ml)			Total K^+=
Potassium Phosphate Inj.(10 mmol K^+/5 mmol Po_4/10 ml)			
10% Calcium Gluconate (2.25 mmol Ca/10 ml)			Total Calories=
50% Magnesium Sulphate (4 mmol/2 ml)			
Zinc Sulphate (50 µmol/ml)			Cal: N_2 Ratio
Addamel (10 ml)			
Solivito (1 vial); Multibionta (10 ml)			Total Volume
Parenterovite			ml
Folic Acid (15 mg/ampoule)			(set on pump)
Vitlipid (A.D.K. –10 ml) add to Intralipid			Infusion Rate
Intralipid –10%/20% – separate/in bag			
Heparin units			ml/hr
Insulin (Actrapid) units			(set on pumps)

Prescriber's Signature   Date Prescribed:

Pharmacist's Signature   Bag Batch N^o :

Fig. 8.8   Central Middlesex Hospital parenteral nutrition prescription sheet.

bag parenteral nutrition prescription sheet which is routinely used throughout the hospital. The prescription is ordered by the physician primarily responsible for the nutritional care of the patient. As several patients may be receiving parenteral nutrition at any one time, is is advisable that the prescription should be submitted to the pharmacy the day before it is needed by the patient, and prescriptions for all weekend requirements should reach the pharmacy before midday on Friday.

Although we are satisfied that fat-emulsion-based parenteral nutrition mixtures are stable for 24 hours, we have not at the time of writing completed our 48 and 72 hour stability studies, so the energy source of our weekend parenteral nutrition mixtures is based on the use of dextrose alone.

Alternative delivery systems

The pharmacy conditions in many hospitals are not suited to the use of the single bag delivery system and alternative regimes have to be designed. As long as the nutritional requirements of the individual patient are assessed carefully and nitrogen and energy sources infused simultaneously, then a three container system can be used, based upon the simultaneous infusion of nitrogen and energy [109].

The solutions are infused through a triple-lead giving set. The Travenol FKC 0181 triple infusion set is recommended because it does not contain an injection site or a stop-cock. Moreover, the leads are joined close to the luer-lock, with lead 1 closest of all. The reason the latter design is an advantage is related to the use of fat emulsions in the system. Fat emulsions have a lower specific gravity than amino acid solutions (Intralipid 20% 0.989; Synthamin 14 1.035). If there is insufficient pressure and insufficient flow rate in the amino acid infusion set, the fat emulsion will flow up into the amino acid solution, a problem that is largely circumvented by the short common arm of the Travenol triple-lead giving set [105].

Three different regimes, suitable for patients with low, intermediate and higher energy and nitrogen requirements are summarised in Fig. 8.9. For all three regimes, the clinician would be advised to commence the infusion at midday to avoid having to change the bottles over when new nursing staff have just arrived on the ward.

Regime A, suitable for patients with low nitrogen requirements, is based upon the daily infusion of 9 g nitrogen.

Three 500 ml bottles containing Intralipid 10%, Synthamin 9 and electrolyte solution A are infused simultaneously over a 12

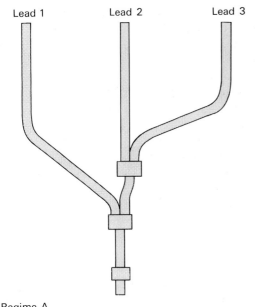

Lead 1	Lead 2	Lead 3

Regime A

Lead 1	Lead 2	Lead 3	Duration
Intralipid 10%	Synthamin 9	Electrolyte A	12 hours
Dextrose 20%	Synthamin 9	Electrolyte B	12 hours

Regime B

Lead 1	Lead 2	Lead 3	Duration
Intralipid 20%	Synthamin 14	Electrolyte A	12 hours
Dextrose 50%	Synthamin 14	Electrolyte B	12 hours

Regime C

Lead 1	Lead 2	Lead 3	Duration
Intralipid 20%	Synthamin 17	Electrolyte A	12 hours
Dextrose 50%	Synthamin 17	Electrolyte B	12 hours

Fig. 8.9. Diagrammatic representation of a three container parenteral nutrition system, describing the use of regimes A, B or C, which are applicable to patients with low, intermediate and higher nitrogen and energy requirements respectively. Vitamin, trace element and insulin supplements are also shown.

hour period through leads 1, 2 and 3 respectively. To prevent mixing, Intralipid must be infused via lead 1. Twelve hours later, preferably at midnight, the empty bottles in leads 1, 2 and 3 are replaced respectively with 500 ml bottles containing dextrose 20%, Synthamin 9 and electrolyte B, and infused over a further 12 hour period. After the completed 24 hour cycle, the giving set is changed (at midday) and the cycle is repeated. For safety, the three bottles for the first 12 hour infusion period are connected to the giving set under sterile conditions in the pharmacy. This regime has been devised so that the non-protein energy to nitrogen ratio (kcal/g N) is approximately 200:1.

The fat-soluble vitamin requirements (1 vial Vitlipid, Table 8.9) are added to the bottle of 10% Intralipid in lead 1. The water soluble vitamin requirements are added to the 20% dextrose in lead 1 (Solivito 1 vial; Multibionta 1 vial; Parentrovite IVHP, ampoules 1 and 2 (Table 8.9), rotated on a daily basis). As mentioned previously, B vitamins are adversely affected by sunlight so the 20% dextrose bottle in lead 1 should be covered by an opaque plastic bag. Trace element supplements (Addamel, 1 vial (Table 8.8)) are added to electrolyte A in lead 3.

Regime B is based on the daily infusion of 14 g nitrogen and maintenance of approximately the same non-protein energy to nitrogen ratio in the first 12 hour period is by substitution of 10% Intralipid in lead 1 with 20% Intralipid, and in the second 12 hour period 20% dextrose in lead 1 is substituted with 50% dextrose. Vitamin and trace element supplements are added as shown in Fig. 8.9. In our experience it has usually been necessary to add insulin supplements to the 50% dextrose (10–30 units of soluble insulin depending on extent of glycosuria and blood glucose levels).

Regime C is based on the use of Synthamin 17, and is suitable for patients with higher energy and nitrogen requirements. The non-protein energy to nitrogen ratio in this regime is lower (159:1) than the ratio in regimes A and B.

Prescription for the regime

In order to assist the nursing staff the author has designed a prescription sheet for the three container delivery system that is identical to Fig. 8.9, except that only one of the regimes A, B or C is listed. The main advantage of such a sheet, as compared to prescribing on the drug sheet, is that it emphasises the importance of making sure that the container connected to lead 1 contains the fat emulsion.

3 litre bag parenteral nutrition mixtures 'to order'

Recently Travenol Laboratories (Caxton Way, Thetford, Norfolk IP24 3SE; Thetford (0842) 4581) have established a new service for hospital pharmacists, whereby parenteral nutrition mixtures prescribed by the clinician are made up into 3 litre containers in the Travenol Compounding Unit, and delivered by them to the hospital pharmacy. Designed primarily as a service to patients on home parenteral nutrition, the service could in the future prove to be of value to hospitals who, for various reasons, do not have laminar flow conditions under which to prepare nutrition mixtures in a single bag container.

Over and underhydration

Probably the most common complications of intravenous fluid management in general are overhydration and underhydration, usually the result of carelessness in the management of fluid balance and inaccurate calculations of the day-to-day gains and losses of fluid [25].

Care should be taken in interpreting rapid gains in weight, especially during the early course of parenteral nutrition, as careful analysis of the fluid balance chart may show, for example, an inescapable correlation between a 1 kg/day weight gain and a

Table 8.11   Metabolic complications of parenteral nutrition.

Hyperglycaemia
Rebound hypoglycaemia and hyperkalaemia
Deficiencies of
    Potassium
    Sodium
    Phosphate
    Zinc
    Magnesium
    Other trace metals
    Folate
    Essential fatty acids
    Vitamins
Osteomalacia
Hypercalcaemia with osteomalacia*
Metabolic acidosis
    Excess amino acids
    Fructose
Increased carbon dioxide production with
    high glucose loads
Hyperammonaemia

Hepatic disturbances
Elevated liver enzymes
Jaundice
Intrahepatic cholestasis
Biliary sludging
Fatty infiltration
Periportal lymphocytic infiltration

Increased gastric acid secretion†

---

* Long-term parenteral nutrition
† There is no evidence of increased erosive gastritis or haemorrhage

1 litre positive water balance, which if it continues will cause major problems.

Glucose intolerance

Catecholamine secretion occurs in response to stress, pain, major trauma and shock [110] and may remain high for some time, dependent on the severity of the injury [111]. Insulin secretion is inhibited by the high catecholamine concentrations [112] so insulin secretion in response to a parenterally administered glucose load may be impaired [6]. Moreover, not only does the pancreas secrete less insulin, but peripheral insulin resistance can be a feature of severe injury [113]. In one large series, 15% of patients receiving parenteral nutrition developed a blood glucose level greater than 400 mg per 100 ml [6]. Furthermore, technical problems of infusions resulted in 9.5% of the patients in the same series developing an episode of hypoglycaemia (blood glucose < 50 mg per 100 ml).

In practical terms, if the patient has 3 + or 4 + glycosuria and a blood glucose above 14 mmol/l he will require insulin. There is controversy as to the route of administration. Thus, insulin administration via an infusion pump, the subcutaneous adminis-tration of soluble insulin or addition of soluble insulin to the dextrose containers have all been advocated. Insulin adheres to the side of most containers, so it may be difficult to judge the correct dose using this route of administration. Despite this, the addition of 1 unit of soluble insulin to each 10 g dextrose in solution will often adequately control blood glucose levels.

If glycosuria is associated with hypokalaemia, then potassium additives (up to 200 mmol/day) alone may correct the problem.

Intracellular ion deficiencies

During the 'flow' phase of injury, loss of intracellular protein carries with it associated intracellular ions. Failure to supplement regimens appropriately can result in deficiency states which usually become overt when the flow phase gives way to anabolism. Thus, potassium, phosphate, zinc, magnesium and folate in serum can fall to dangerously low levels. Potassium losses usually occur in a fixed ratio to nitrogen losses, and a patient in negative nitrogen balance develops a deficiency of 3 mmol potassium for every gram of nitrogen lost [114]. Hypophos-phataemia can result in rapid onset of dysarthria, paraesthesiae, disorientation, coma and asthenia (including impairment of respiratory muscle function). Decreases in red cell 2,3-diphos-phoglycerate shift the oxygen dissociation curve to the left and red cell ATP may fall to 15% of normal.

Zinc deficiency

Although low serum zinc levels do not necessarily imply a total body or intracellular deficiency, falling levels should be covered by increased zinc supplements, as mentioned in Chapter 6. Zinc deficiency causes diarrhoea, impaired insulin responses, leucocyte function and wound healing, and in addition a positive nitrogen balance cannot be achieved. Cutaneous manifestations resemble perioral and perineal candidiasis and also include stomatitis, alopecia, increased pigmentation and an acrodermatitis enteropathica-like dermatitis.

Magnesium deficiency

Magnesium deficiency may induce muscular fibrillation and should be suspected in patients with prolonged diarrhoea (e.g. Crohn's disease) or resistant hypokalaemia.

Other deficiencies

As mentioned previously in Chapter 6, deficiencies of a number of trace elements have been described during parenteral nutrition (e.g. copper, cobalt, selenium, manganese and molybdenum). Unfortunately, knowledge of requirements during parenteral nutrition is limited and it is not possible to routinely measure either tissue or circulating levels.

Vitamin deficiency
Vitamin deficiencies tend to occur under similar circumstances to intracellular ion deficiencies. Thiamine deficiency in alcoholics may be unmasked by carbohydrate infusions, thus precipitating acute Wernicke's encephalopathy with coma. Folate depletion occurs rapidly in catabolic patients during parenteral nutrition in the absence of folate supplementation and may lead to acute pancytopenia, jaundice and impaired protein synthesis by interference with methionine metabolism [115]. Vitamins A and K should be given, but the position of vitamin D is currently a subject of review. Unless vitamin D deficiency or a condition likely to cause it is present before parenteral nutrition is started, supplement of this vitamin is not indicated for short-term parenteral nutrition.

Bone disease associated with parenteral nutrition

Although long-term parenteral nutrition has led to overt rickets and osteomalacia, sometimes requiring high doses of vitamin D for correction [116], a further syndrome has been described which includes hypercalcaemia, hypercalcuria, hyperphosphaturia and abnormal parathyroid hormone levels in conjunction with clinical and histological pictures resembling osteomalacia [117]. It has been suggested that such changes may result from excess phosphate and vitamin D administration [118].

Liver function test changes

Abnormal liver function tests frequently occur during parenteral nutrition [119]. A cholestatic picture tends to predominate, with rises in alkaline phosphatase and bilirubin. Elevations in serum transaminases may, however, also be seen. Liver biopsies performed in our patients show histological evidence of fatty infiltration, periportal lymphocytic infiltration with bile duct proliferation and intrahepatic cholestasis, or biliary sludging resulting in extrahepatic obstruction.

A great deal of speculation surrounds the causes of these biochemical and histological abnormalities. Rises in alkaline phosphatase, minimal changes in transaminases and fatty infiltration may be due to underlying protein-calorie malnutrition *per se* or to the use of nutrition regimes based on excessively high non-protein energy to nitrogen ratios (> 200 kcal/g) [120].

Ultrasound examinations show that all patients are likely to develop sludge in the gallbladder after seven weeks parenteral nutrition [121], which is likely to explain the other histological abnormalities seen, as well as the clinical cholestatic jaundice that a few of these patients develop. Although the mechanisms underlying these changes are also unknown, they are rapidly reversible on stopping parenteral nutrition [121].

In our experience none of the biochemical abnormalities in the anicteric patient have any significant clinical consequence, and are rapidly reversible after parenteral nutrition is discontinued.

Finally, it is important to remember that co-existing underlying medical problems rather than parentral nutrition may be responsible for the liver function test changes. If, however, a patient on parenteral nutrition becomes jaundiced, and extrahepatic obstruction due to biliary sludging is thought to be responsible, cyclic (nocturnal) parenteral nutrition [122] should be tried, as there is some evidence that reversal of abnormalities of liver function may follow replacement of continuous parenteral nutrition with cyclic parenteral nutrition [123].

PATIENT MONITORING (Table 8.12)

There is a clear need to carefully monitor treatment in patients

Table **8.12** Patient monitoring.

Parameters	Before treatment	Daily	Twice weekly	Weekly
Weight	✓			✓
Mid triceps skinfold thickness	✓		✓	
Arm muscle circumference	✓			✓
Serum albumin	✓			✓
Serum transferrin	✓			✓
Lymphocyte count	✓			✓
Skin tests for Candida				
PPD (tuberculin)				
Streptokinase				
Streptodornase				
FBP ESR	✓		✓	
Serum iron	✓			✓
Folic acid	✓			✓
Vitamin B12	✓			✓
Prothrombin time	✓			✓
Blood glucose*	✓	✓		
Urinary glucose*		✓		
Electrolytes and urea*	✓	✓		
Calcium	✓		✓	
Phosphate	✓		✓	
Magnesium	✓		✓	
Zinc	✓		✓	
Liver function tests	✓	✓		
24 hour urinary urea excretion (for nitrogen balance estimations)				

* Depending on clinical and biochemical state of the patient

needing parenteral nutrition. Table 8.12 outlines the simple ways of monitoring nutritional status and immune response (weight, triceps skinfold thickness, arm muscle circumference, serum albumin, lymphocyte count and possibly delayed hypersensitivity skin testing).

As part of our initial assessment of nutritional status these parameters are routinely measured before treatment and our usual practice is to assess changes at weekly or two-weekly intervals during parenteral nutrition.

In view of the frequency of the metabolic problems that can occur in patients on parenteral nutrition, due both to the underlying disease process as well as parenteral nutrition *per se*, frequent measurements of urinary glucose, blood glucose, electrolytes and urea, creatinine, calcium, phosphate, magnesium, zinc and liver function tests should all be performed. The recommendations in Table 8.12 should be considered as guidelines only, and more frequent measurements may be required. In general, the management of the sick patient on parenteral nutrition requires the same approach as that adopted for the management of any patient in an intensive care unit.

ENDING PARENTERAL NUTRITION

When a planned course of parenteral nutrition is discontinued, it is quite likely that the patient will require enteral feeding. If so, the principles outlined in the previous chapter should be adhered to. As far as possible, the changeover should be gradual, with the infusion rate of the parenteral regime being slowed over two to three days while the enteral nutrition regime is gradually being introduced. This is because patients who have received parenteral nutrition for prolonged periods of time will have a reduced appetite and are at particular risk of developing diarrhoea on oral or tube feeding regimes.

In practice what often happens is that the decision to discontinue parenteral nutrition may be forced (commonly on account of purely technical problems) when the patient is in the anabolic phase of the response to injury, in positive nitrogen balance and improving. This being the case, patients may not need to receive enteral nutrition and can be started on a light diet, this in turn being changed to normal food as soon as possible.

HOME PARENTERAL NUTRITION

Patients with short bowel syndrome, extensive Crohn's disease and other irreversible causes of malabsorption (who would otherwise die or survive in a grossly malnourished state) can now be managed on home parenteral nutrition. It goes without saying that before embarking on home parenteral nutrition all efforts to maintain the patient on enteral nutrition must have failed.

In England and Wales it is probable that there are no more than 20 patients on home parenteral nutrition at any one time [124]. In the USA, however, it has been suggested that there may be as many as 300 [125].

In this country, Crohn's disease appears to be the commonest indication for treatment [124], the individual indications varying from extensive disease to multiple fistulas and the short bowel syndrome after extensive resection. The basic principle is to infuse nutrients intravenously during a 10–12 hour overnight period to approximate daily requirements, while encouraging patients to pursue normal activities during the day [125]. There is general agreement that home parenteral nutrition is best administered into the subclavian vein through a subcutaneously tunnelled silicone rubber catheter with the tip positioned in the superior vena cava [124].

The importance of adequate home conditions and catheter care must be stressed, and account must be taken of the ability of the patient and relatives to understand the treatment. The degree of success achieved by patients in managing this treatment has been shown by the virtually universal finding that catheter-related sepsis rates are lower when patients receive parenteral nutrition at home than in hospital [124].

The active participation of specialised nursing staff, dietitians, pharmacists and the medical team is essential [124], and one report from America has highlighted the importance of the social worker in overall patient care [126].

PROTEIN-SPARING THERAPY— PERIPHERAL ISOTONIC AMINO ACID INFUSION

Blackburn and co-workers have recently shown that the peripheral venous administration of isotonic amino acid solutions has a significant preservative effect on nitrogen balance in a group of stressed patients compared to similar patients treated with 5% dextrose therapy [89, 127, 128]. In these studies [89], blood glucose and insulin levels were lower in the amino acid- than dextrose-treated group; in contrast levels of ketone bodies (acetoacetate + β-OH butyric acid) and free fatty acids were higher in the amino acid-treated group. Based upon these findings, Blackburn has suggested that whereas the insulin response to glucose infusion stimulates protein catabolism by virtue of depressing lipolysis, amino acid infusion has no antilipolytic or antiketogenic effect, thereby diminishing the protein catabolic response to injury [89, 127, 128].

Others have now confirmed Blackburn's observations showing that significant nitrogen sparing can be achieved with isotonic amino acid solutions in the post-operative period [129–132]. There is disagreement, however, about the mechanisms involved. Thus both Greenberg *et al* [84] and Rowlands and Clark [133] have failed to substantiate the claims that the beneficial effect is in any way related to the degree of fat mobilisation.

Given that the metabolic advantages of peripheral isotonic amino acid therapy are clear in terms of nitrogen balance, the most important question that remains is whether this type of therapy has any significant clinical advantages over conventional dextrose and saline solutions that have been the main method of feeding patients who are unlikely to require nutritional support. Two carefully designed controlled trials definitely suggest that it does not [134, 135]. Sagar, however [136] has shown that patients in his treatment group were discharged from hospital earlier than the control patients, but this can hardly be heralded as a significant clinical advance. Until such time as controlled trials show significant benefits of this novel therapeutic approach to nutritional support, we continue to treat our post-operative patients with a mixture of 5% dextrose and saline until it becomes evident to us that either enteral or standard central venous nutrition is indicated.

REFERENCES

1   Welch G.W., McKell D.W., Silverstein P., *et al* (1974) The role of catheter composition in the development of thrombophlebitis. *Surg. Gynaec. Obstet.* **138**, 421.

2   Jones B.J.M. & Silk D.B.A. (1982) Parenteral nutrition. *Med. Int.* **1**, 674.

3   Dudrick S.J., Wilmore D.W., Vars H.M. & Rhoads J.E. (1968) Long-term parenteral nutrition with growth, development and positive nitrogen balance. *Surgery* **64**, 134.

4   Dudrick S.J., Wilmore D.W., Vars H.M. & Rhoads J.E. (1969) Can intravenous feeding as the sole means of nutrition support growth in the child and restore weight loss in an adult? An affirmative answer. *Ann. Surg.* **169**, 974.

5   Ryan J.A., Abel R.M., Abbott W.M., *et al* (1974) Catheter complications in total parenteral nutrition: a prospective study of 200 consecutive patients. *New Engl. J. Med.* **290**, 757.

6   Ryan J.A. (1976) Complications of total parenteral nutrition. In

Total Parenteral Nutrition, ed. J.E. Fischer, p. 55. Little Brown, Boston.

7 Bernard R.W. & Stahl W.M. (1971) Subclavian vein catheterisation. A prospective study: 1. Noninfectious complications. *Ann. Surg.* **173**, 184.

8 Walter C.W. (1978) Bacterial contamination of intravenous infusion due to faulty technique. In *Advances in Parenteral Nutrition*, ed. I.D.A. Johnston, p. 325. MTP Press, Lancaster.

9 Powell-Tuck J. (1978) Skin tunnel for central venous catheter: non-operative techniques. *Br. Med. J.* **1**, 625.

10 Powell-Tuck J., Nielsen T., Farwell J.A. & Lennard-Jones J.E. (1978) Team approach to long-term intravenous feeding in patients with gastrointestinal disorders. *Lancet* **ii**, 825.

11 Powell-Tuck J., Lennard-Jones J.E., Lowes J.A., *et al* (1979) Intravenous feeding in a Gastroenterological Unit. A prospective study of infective complications. *J. Clin. Pathol.* **32**, 549.

12 Curry C.R. & Quie P.G. (1971) Fungal septicaemia in patients receiving parenteral hyperalimentation. *New Engl. J. Med.* **285**, 1221.

13 Parsa M.H., Habif D.V., Ferrer J.M., *et al* (1972) Intravenous hyperalimentation: Indications, technique and complications. *Bull. NY Acad. Med.* **48**, 920.

14 Keohane P.P., Attrill H., Jones B.J.M., Northover J., Cribb A. & Silk D.B.A. (1983) Significance of tunnelling and a nutrition nurse in TPN catheter sepsis—a controlled trial. *J. Parent. Ent. Nutr.* (in press).

15 Jarrard M.M. & Freeman J.B. (1976) The effects of antibiotic ointments and antiseptics on the skin flora beneath subclavian catheters during intravenous hyperalimentation. *J. Surg. Res.* **22**, 521.

16 Philipps K.J. (1976) Nursing care in parenteral nutrition. In *Total Parenteral Nutrition*, ed. J.E. Fischer, p. 101. Little Brown, Boston.

17 McLean Ross A.H., Anderson J.R. & Walls A.D.F. (1980) Central venous catheterisation. *Ann. Roy. Coll. Surg. Eng.* **62**, 454.

18 McLean Ross A.H., Griffith C.D.M., Anderson J.R. & Grieve D.C. (1982) Thromboembolic complications with silicone elastomer subclavian catheters. *J. Parent. Ent. Nutr.* **6**, 61.

19 Popp M.D., Law E.J. & MacMillan B.G. (1974) Parenteral nutrition in the burned child. A study of 26 patients. *Ann. Surg.* **179**, 219.

20 Warden G.D., Wilmore D. & Pruitt B.A. (1973) Central vein thrombosis: a hazard of medical progress. *J. Trauma* **13**, 620.

21 Valerio D., Hussey J.K. & Smith F.W. (1981) Central venous thrombosis associated with intravenous feeding—a prospective study. *J. Parent. Ent. Nutr.* **5**, 240.

22 Stein J.M. & Pruitt B.A. (1970) Suppurative thrombophlebitis—a lethal iatrogenic disease. *New Engl. J. Med.* **282**, 1452.

23 Bailey M.J. (1979) Reduction of catheter-associated sepsis in parenteral nutrition using low dose intravenous heparin. *Br. Med. J.* **1**, 1671.

24 Collin J., Tweedle D.E.F., Venables C.W., *et al* (1973) Effect of a millipore filter on complications of intravenous infusions: a prospective clinical trial. *Br. Med. J.* **4**, 456.

25 Wright P.D. (1980) Problems in intravenous therapy. *J. Roy. Coll. Phys. Lond.* **14**, 161.

26 Flanagan J.P., Gradisar I.A., Gross R.J. & Kelly T.R. (1969) Air embolus—a lethal complication of subclavian venipuncture. *New Engl. J. Med.* **281**, 488.

27 Green H.L. & Nemir P. (1971) Air embolism as a complication during parenteral alimentation. *Am. J. Surg.* **121**, 164.

28 Paskin D.L., Hoffman W.S. & Tuddenham W.J. (1974) A new complication of subclavian vein catheterisation. *Ann. Surg.* **179**, 266.

29 Allen J.R. (1978) The incidence of nosocomial infection in patients receiving total parenteral nutrition. In *Advances in Parenteral Nutrition* (Ed Johnston I.D.A.), p. 339. MTP Press, Lancaster.

30 Wilmore D.W., Groff D.B., Bishop H.C. & Dudrick S.J. (1969) Total parenteral nutrition in infants with catastrophic gastrointestinal anomalies. *J. Ped. Surg.* **4**, 181.

31 Boeckman C.R. & Krill C.E. (1970) Bacterial and fungal infections complicating parenteral alimentation in infants and children. *J. Ped. Surg.* **5**, 117.

32 Sanders R.A. & Sheldon G.F. (1976) Septic complications of total parenteral nutrition. *Am. J. Surg.* **132**, 214.

33 Jones B.J.M., Keohane P.P. & Silk D.B.A. (1982) Personal observation.

34 Myers R.N., Smink R.D. & Goldstein F. (1974) Parenteral hyperalimentation—five years' clinical experience. *Am. J. Gastroenterol.* **62**, 313.

35 Powell C., Regan C., Fabri P.J. & Ruberg R.L. (1982) Evaluation of opsite catheter dressings for parenteral nutrition: a prospective, randomised study. *J. Parent. Ent. Nutr.* **6**, 43.

36 Norden C.W. (1969) Application of antibiotic ointment to the site of venous catheterisation—a controlled trial. *J. Infect. Dis.* **120**, 611.

37 Maki D.G., Rhame F.S., Mackel D.C. & Bennett J.V. (1976) Nationwide epidemic of septicaemia caused by contaminated intravenous products. 1. Epidemiologic and clinical features. *Am. J. Med.* **60**, 471.

38 Buxton A.E., Highsmith A.K., Garner J.S., *et al* (1979) Contamination of intravenous fluid: effects of changing administration sets. *Ann. Int. Med.* **90**, 764.

39 Dillon J.D., Schaffner W., Van Way C.W. & Meng H.C. (1973) Septicaemia and total parenteral nutrition: distinguishing catheter-related from other septic episodes. *J. Am. Med. Assoc.* **223**, 1341.

40 Goldstein E. & Hoeprich P.D. (1972) Problems in the diagnosis and treatment of systemic candidiasis. *J. Infect. Dis.* **125**, 190.

41 Sim A.J.W., Wolfe B.M., Young V.R., *et al* (1979) Glucose promotes whole body protein synthesis from infused amino acids in fasting man. *Lancet* **i**, 68.

42 Tweedle D.E.F. (1973) The effect of amino acid solutions of differing composition in the nitrogen balance of post-operative patients. *J. Roy. Coll. Surg. Edin.* **18**, 580.

43 Tweedle D.E.F., Spivey J. & Johnston I.D.A. (1973) Choice of intravenous amino acid solutions for use after surgical operations. *Metabolism* **22**, 173.

44 Hartley T.F. & Lee H.A. (1975) Investigations into the optimum nitrogen and calorie requirements and comparative nutritive value of three intravenous amino acid solutions in the post-operative period. *Nutr. Metab.* **19**, 201.

45 Anonymous (1980) Adult parenteral nutrition: Which preparations? *Drug Ther. Bull.* **18**, 85.

46 Jackson A.A. & Golder M.H.N. (1980) ^{15}N Glycine metabolism in normal man: the metabolic amino-nitrogen pool. *Clin. Sci.* **58**, 517.

47 Batstone G.F., Gent A.E. & Shakespeare P.G. (1981) Cost-effective parenteral feeding. *Lancet* **i**, 225.

48 Allison S.P., Hinton P. & Chamberlain M.J. (1968) Intravenous glucose tolerance, insulin and free fatty acid levels in burned patients. *Lancet* **ii**, 1113.

49 Zollner N. (1978) Evaluation of non-glucose carbohydrates in parenteral nutrition. In *Advances in Parenteral Nutrition*, ed. I.D.A. Johnston, p. 61. MTP Press, Lancaster.

50 Weischelbaum T.E., Margraf H.W. & Elman R. (1953) Metabolism of intravenously infused fructose in man. *Metabolism* **2**, 434.

51 Topping D.L. & Mayes P.A. (1972) The immediate effects of insulin and fructose on the metabolism of the perfused liver. *Biochem J.* **126**, 295.

52 Miller M., Craig J.W., Drucker W.R. & Woodward H. (1956) The metabolism of fructose in man. *Yale. J. Biol. Med.* **29**, 335.

53 Thoren L. (1962) Parenteral nutrition with carbohydrate and alcohol. *Acta. Chir. Scand.* **325**, 75.

54 Bergstom J. & Hulfman E. (1967) Synthesis of muscle glycogen in man after glucose and fructose infusion. *Acta Med. Scand.* **182**, 93.

55 Burch H.B., Lowry O.H., Meinhardt L., Max P. & Chyu K. (1970) Effect of fructose, dihydroxy acetone, glycerol and glucose on metabolism and related compounds in liver and kidney. *J. Biol. Chem.* **245**, 2092.

56 Woods H.F., Eggleston L.V. & Krebs H.A. (1970) The cause of hepatic accumulation of fructose-1-phosphate on fructose loading. *Biochem. J.* **119**, 501.

57 Sestoft L., Tonnesen K., Hansen F.V. & Damgaard S.E. (1972) Fructose and D-glyceraldehyde metabolism in the isolated perfused pig liver. *Eur. J. Biochem.* **30**, 542.

58 Maenpaa P.H., Raivo K.O. & Kekomaki M.P. (1968) Liver adenine nucleotides: fructose induced depletion and its effect on protein synthesis. *Science* **161**, 1253.

59 Bassler K.H. (1976) Quantitative aspects of the metabolism of glucose, fructose, sorbitol and xylitol. In *Monosaccharides and Polyalcohols in Nutrition; Therapy and Dietetics*, eds. G. Ritzel and G. Brubacher, p. 22. Hans Huber, Bern.

60 Heuckenkamp P.U. (1976) Comparison of glucose, fructose and xylitol for parenteral alimentation in metabolically healthy men. In *Monosaccharides and Polyalcohols in Nutrition, Therapy and Dietetics*, eds. G. Ritzel and G. Brubacher, p. 170. Hans Huber, Bern.

61 Woods H.F. & Krebs H.A. (1971) Lactate production in the perfused rat liver. *Biochem. J.* **125**, 129.

62 Newton D., Connor H. & Woods H.F. (1978) Metabolic pathways

for carbohydrates in parenteral nutrition. In *Advances in Parenteral Nutrition*, ed. I.D.A. Johnston, p. 29. MTP Press, Lancaster.

63 Cohen R.D. & Woods H.F. (1976) *Clinical and Biochemical Aspects of Lactic Acidosis*, p. 194, Blackwell Scientific Publications, Oxford.

64 Bassler K.H., Stein G. & Belzer W. (1966) Xylistoffwechsel und xylitresorption stoffwechsel-adaptation als ursache fur lesorptions beschleunigtng. *Biochem. J.* **246**, 171.

65 Jacob A., Williamson J.R. & Asakura T. (1971) Xylitol metabolism in perfused rat liver. *J. Biol. Chem.* **246**, 7623.

66 Lee H.A. (1978) Parenteral nutrition. In *Nutrition in Clinical Management of Disease*, eds. J.W.T. Dickerson and H.A. Lee. Edward Arnold, London.

67 Bickel H., Matzkies F., Fekl W. & Berg G. (1973) Verwertung und stoffwechselverhal ten von sorbit wahrend paventeraler langzei-tinfusion. *Dtsch. Med. Wschr.* **98**, 2079.

68 Muller F., Strack E., Kuhfahl E. & Dettmer D. (1967) Der stoffwechsel von xylit bei normalen und alloxamdiabetischen kaninchen. *Z. ges. exp. Med.* **142**, 338.

69 Young J.M. & Weser E. (1971) The metabolism of circulating maltose in man. *J. Clin. Invest.* **50**, 986.

70 Sprandel U., Henckenkamp P.U. & Zollner N. (1975) Utilisation of intravenous maltose. *Nutr. Metab.* **19**, 96.

71 Finke C. & Reinauer H. (1976) Uber den Abban von infundierter Maltose beim Menschen. *Ernahrungswiss* **15**, 231.

72 Bibby R.J., Davies D. & Mallick N.P. (1974) Studies of the metabolism of dextrin, Caloreen, administered intravenously in human subjects. *Clin. Sci. Mol. Med.* **46**, 7P.

73 Young G.A., Fletcher J.T., Cioletti L.A., *et al* (1981) Metabolism of parenteral glucose oligosaccharide in man. *J. Parent. Ent. Nutr.* **5**, 369.

74 Meng H.C. (1976) Fat emulsions in parenteral nutrition. In *Total Parenteral Nutrition*, ed. J.E. Fischer, p. 305. Little Brown, Boston.

75 Hallberg D. (1965) Studies on the elimination of exogenous lipids from the blood stream: kinetics for the elimination of a fat emulsion studied by a single injection technique in man. *Acta Physiol. Scand.* **64**, 304.

76 Goffe G., Jacobson S. & Wretlind A. (1976) Lipid emulsions and technique of peripheral administration in parenteral nutrition. In *Total Parenteral Nutrition* ed J.E. Fischer, p. 335. Little Brown, Boston.

77 Scow R.O. (1970) Transport of triglyceride: its removal from blood circulation and uptake by tissues. In *Parenteral Nutrition*, eds. H.C. Meng and D.H. Law, p. 194. C. Thomas, Springfield, Illinois.

78 Scow R.O., Hamosh M., Blanchette-Mackie J. & Evans A.J. (1972) Uptake of blood triglyceride by various tissues. *Lipids* **7**, 497.

79 Boberg J., Carlson L.A. & Hallberg D. (1969) Application of a new intravenous fat tolerance test in the study of hypertriglyceridaemia in man. *J. Athero. Scl. Res.* **9**, 159.

80 Jeejeebhoy K.N., Anderson G.H., Nakhoods A.F., Greenberg G.R., Sanderson I. & Marliss E.B. (1976) Metabolic studies in total nutrition with lipid in man. *J. Clin. Invest.* **57**, 125.

81 Bark S., Holm I., Hakansson I., *et al* (1976) Nitrogen sparing effect

of fat emulsion compared with glucose in the post-operative period. *Acta Chir. Scand.* **142**, 423.

82 Gazzaniga A.B., Bartlett R.H. & Shobe J.B. (1975) Nitrogen balance in patients receiving either fat or carbohydrate for total parenteral nutrition. *Ann. Surg.* **182**, 163.

83 Broviac J.N., Riella M.C. & Scribner B.H. (1976) The role of Intralipid in prolonged parenteral nutrition. 1. As a calorie substitute for glucose. *Am. J. Clin. Nutr.* **29**, 255.

84 Greenberg G.R., Marliss E.B., Anderson G.H., Langer B., Spence W. *et al* (1976) Protein sparing therapy in post-operative patients: effects of added hypocaloric glucose or lipid. *New Engl. J. Med.* **294**, 1411.

85 Macfie J., Smith R.C. & Hill G.L. (1981) Glucose or fat as a non-protein energy source? A controlled trial in gastroenterological patients requiring parenteral nutrition. *Gastroenterology* **80**, 103.

86 Holliday R.L., Viidik T. & Jennings B. (1978) Lipid metabolism in stress. In *Advances in Parenteral Nutrition*, ed. I.D.A. Johnston, p. 179. MTP Press, Lancaster.

87 Clowes G.H., O'Donnell T.F., Ryan N.T. & Blackburn G.L. (1974) Energy metabolism in sepsis. *Ann. Surg.* **179**, 684.

88 O'Donnell T.F., Clowes G.H., Blackburn G.L., *et al* (1976) Proteolysis associated with a deficit of peripheral energy fuel substrates in septic man. *Surgery* **80**, 191.

89 Blackburn G.L., Pratt J.P. & Hensle T.W. (1976) Peripheral amino acid infusions. In *Total Parenteral Nutrition*, ed. J.E. Fischer, p. 363. Little Brown, Boston.

90 Long J.M., Wilmore D.W., Mason A.D. & Pruitt B.A. (1977) Effect of carbohydrate and fat intake on nitrogen excretion during intravenous feeding. *Ann. Surg.* **185**, 417.

91 McDougall W.S., Wilmore D.W. & Pruitt B.A. (1977) Effect of neat isosmotic intravenous nutrient infusions on nitrogen balance in critically ill injured patients. *Surg. Gynaecol. Obstet.* **145**, 408.

92 Long J.M., Wilmore D.W., Mason A.D., *et al* (1974) Fat carbohydrate interaction. Effects on nitrogen sparing in total intravenous feeding. *Surg. Forum.* **25**, 61.

93 Allison S.P. (1980) Effect of insulin on metabolic response to injury. *J. Parent. Ent. Nutr.* **4**, 175.

94 Askanazi J., Carpentier Y.A., Elwyn D.H., *et al* (1980) Influence of total parenteral nutrition on fuel utilisation in injury and sepsis. *Ann. Surg.* **191**, 40.

95 Burr G.O. & Burr M.M. (1929) A new deficiency disease produced by the rigid exclusion of fat from the diet. *J. Biol. Chem.* **82**, 345.

96 Holman R.T. (1960) The ratio of trienoic:tetraenoic acids in tissue lipids as a measure of essential fatty acid requirement. *J. Nutr.* **70**, 405.

97 Goodgame J.T., Lowry S.F. & Brennan M.F. (1978) Essential fatty acid deficiency in total parenteral nutrition: time course of development and suggestions for therapy. *Surgery* **84**, 271.

98 Dudrick S.J. & Ruberg R.L. (1971) Principles and practice of parenteral nutrition. *Gastroenterology* **61**, 901.

99 Peters C. & Fischer J.E. (1980) Studies on calorie to nitrogen ratio for total parenteral nutrition. *Surg. Gynecol. Obstet.* **151**, 1.

100 Smith R.C., Burkinshaw L. & Hill G.L. (1982) Optimal energy and nitrogen intake for gastroenterological patients requiring parenteral nutrition. *Gastroenterology* **82**, 445.

101 Peters C. & Fischer J.E. (1980) Studies on calorie to nitrogen ratio for total parenteral nutrition. *Surg. Gynaecol. Obstet.* **151**, 1.

102 Sheldon G.F. (1982) Optimal energy and nutritional intake in total parenteral nutrition. *Gastroenterology* **82**, 586.

103 Powell-Tuck J. & Goode A.W. (1981) Principles of enteral and parenteral nutrition. *Br. J. Anaesth.* **53**, 169.

104 Giovanoni R. (1976) The manufacturing pharmacy. Solutions and incompatibilities. In *Total Parenteral Nutrition*, ed. J.E. Fischer, p. 27. Little Brown, Boston.

105 Tweedle D.E.F. (1978) The use of fat emulsions in parenteral nutrition. In *Advances in Parenteral Nutrition*, ed. I.D.A. Johnston, p. 165. MTP Press, Lancaster.

106 Solassol C., Joyeux H., Serrou B., *et al* (1973) Nouvelles Techniques de nutrition parenterale a long terme pour supleance intestinale. *Chirurgie* **105**, 15.

107 Solassol C. & Joyeux H. (1974) Nouvelle techniques pour nutrition parenterale chronique. *Ann. Anaesth. Franc. Special* **2**, 75.

108 Hardy G. & Klim R.A. (1982) Stability studies on parenteral nutrition mixtures with lipids. *J. Parent. Ent. Nutr.* **5**, 569.

109 Silk D.B.A. (1978) Clinical nutrition in hospitals. 3. Parenteral nutrition. *Hosp. Update* **4**, 611.

110 Woolfson A.M.J. (1979) Metabolic considerations in nutritional support. *Res. Clin. Forums* **1**, 35.

111 Birke G., Duner H., Liljedahl S.O., Pernow B., Plantin L.O. & Troelle L. (1957) Histamine, catecholamines and adrenocorticol-steroids in burns. *Acta Chir. Scand.* **114**, 87.

112 Porte D., Graber A.L., Kuzuya T. & Williams R.H. (1966) The effect of epinephrine on immunoreactive insulin levels in man. *J. Clin. Invest.* **45**, 228.

113 Porte D. & Bagdale J.D. (1970) Human insulin secretion: an integrated approach. *Ann. Rev. Med.* **21**, 219.

114 Dudrick S.J., Macfayden B.V., Van Buren C.T., Ruberg R.L. & Maynard A.T. (1972) Parenteral hyperalimentation, metabolic problems and solutions. *Ann. Surg.* **176**, 259.

115 Wardrop C.A.J., Heatley R.V., Tennant G.B., *et al* (1975) Acute folate deficiency in surgical patients on amino acid/ethanol intravenous nutrition. *Lancet* **ii**, 640.

116 Jones B.J.M. & Silk D.B.A. (1982) Parenteral nutrition. *Med. Int.* **1**, 674.

117 Klein G.L., Ament M.E., Bluestone R., *et al* (1980) Bone disease associated with total parenteral nutrition. *Lancet* **ii**, 1041.

118 Allam B.F., Dryburgh F.J. & Shenkin A. (1981) Metabolic bone disease during parenteral nutrition. *Lancet* **i**, 385.

119 Sitges-Crens A., Canadas E. & Vilar L. (1978) Cholestatic jaundice during parenteral alimentation in adults. In *Advances in Parenteral Nutrition*, ed. I.D.A. Johnston, p. 461. MTP Press, Lancaster.

120 Rowlands B.J. & Dudrick S.J. (1982) Gall bladder bile composition during intravenous hyperalimentation in dogs. *J. Parent. Ent. Nutr.* **5**, 577.

121 Messing B., Bories C., Kunstlinger F. & Bernier J.J. (1982) Does parenteral nutrition induce a lithogenic gallbladder bile? *J. Parent. Ent. Nutr.* **5**, 560.

122 Matuchansky C., Morichau-Beauchant M., Druart F. & Tapin J. (1961) Cyclic (nocturnal) total parenteral nutrition in hospitalised adult patients with severe digestive diseases. Report of a prospective study. *Gastroenterology* **81**, 433.

123 Maini B., Blackburn G.L., Bristian B.R., *et al* (1976) Cyclic hyperalimentation: an optimal technique for preservation of visceral protein. *J. Surg. Res.* **20**, 515.

124 Occasional Review—Home parenteral nutrition in England and Wales. Report on a symposium held at Hope Hospital, Salford on 3 July 1980. *Br. Med. J.* **281**, 1407.

125 Fleming C.R., Beart R.W., Berkner S., *et al* (1980) Home parenteral nutrition for management of the severely malnourished adult patient. *Gastroenterology* **79**, 11.

126 Robinovitch A.E. (1981) Home total parenteral nutrition. A psycho-social viewpoint. *J. Parent. Ent. Nutr.* **5**, 522.

127 Blackburn G.L., Flatt J.P., Clowes G.H.A. Jr, *et al* (1973) Protein sparing therapy during periods of starvation with sepsis or trauma. *Ann. Surg.* **177**, 588.

128 Blackburn G.L., Flatt J.P., Clowes G.H.A. Jr, *et al* (1973) Peripheral intravenous feeding with isotonic amino acid solutions. *Am. J. Surg.* **125**, 447.

129 Freeman J.B., Stegink L.D., Meyer P.D., Thompson R.J. & Denbest L. (1975) Metabolic effects of amino acids v dextrose infusion in surgical patients. *Arch. Surg.* **110**, 916.

130 Hoover H.C., Grant J.P., Gorschboth C. & Ketcham A.S. (1975) Nitrogen sparing intravenous fluids in post-operative patients. *New Engl. J. Med.* **293**, 172.

131 Schulte W.J., Condon O.C. & Krans M.A. (1975) Positive nitrogen balance using isotonic crystalline amino acid solutions. *Arch. Surg.* **110**, 914.

132 Gazzaniga A.B., Day A.T., Bartlett R.H. & Wilson A.F. (1976) Endogenous calorie sources and nitrogen balance regulation in post-operative patients. *Arch. Surg.* **111**, 1357.

133 Rowlands B.J. & Clark R.G. (1978) Post-operative amino acid infusions: an appraisal. *Br. J. Surg.* **65**, 384.

134 Collins J.P., Oxby C.B. & Hill G.L. (1978) Intravenous amino acids and intravenous hyperalimentation as protein sparing therapy after major surgery. A controlled clinical trial. *Lancet* **i**, 788.

135 Smith J.A.R., Woods H.F. & Simms J.M. (1981) A comparison of peripheral and central venous nutrition after major abdominal surgery. In *Proceedings 3rd European Congress on Parenteral and Enteral Nutrition*, p. 99.

136 Sagar S. (1980) Peripheral vein isotonic amino acid therapy. *Br. J. Intraven. Ther.*, December, p. 30.

Chapter 9
The Liver and Nutrition

It has been recognised for many years that patients with chronic parenchymal liver disease are malnourished. In a recent report O'Keefe and co-workers have found that on formal testing a significant proportion of their patients exhibited clinical, bio-chemical, haematological and immunological parameters thought to be indicative of protein calorie malnutrition [1], and furthermore their data suggested a link between malnutrition, energy, sepsis and mortality in their patients [1].

The liver plays a central role in the digestion, metabolism and storage of nutrients, and malnutrition probably arises in these patients as a result of the combination of decreased intake, decreased absorption, decreased storage and abnormalities of metabolism [2].

Poor dietary intake is almost certainly one of the principle causes of nutritional deficiencies in chronic liver disease [3, 4]. This may arise on account of associated anorexia and nausea and also because dietary protein intake is often restricted for thera-peutic reasons as part of the management of hepatic encephalo-pathy. Evidence is also accumulating to suggest that nutritional deficiencies arise on account of impaired digestion and absorption of nutrients. To date, pancreatic exocrine insufficiency has been demonstrated in cirrhotic patients [5], as well as malabsorption of D-xylose, thiamine, folic acid and fat [6].

HEPATIC ENCEPHALOPATHY—THE DILEMMA

It is a feature of the natural history of the disease that most patients with hepatic cirrhosis will develop hepatic encephalo-pathy and coma at some stage during the course of their illness. The commonest precipitating causes are infection, electrolyte abnormalities (often caused by diuretic abuse), variceal haemorr-hage, sedative abuse and constipation.

One of the greatest dilemmas in clinical hepatology is that one is often forced to restrict protein intake in an already malnour-ished cirrhotic patient in an attempt to improve or prevent the onset of hepatic encephalopathy. Thus, while the mental state of these patients may improve by dietary protein restriction, their nutritional status may be worsened. This can lead to a vicious circle because malnutrition may be one of the reasons why these patients are unduly susceptible to developing infection and, as is widely known, infection is one of the most common precipitating causes of hepatic encephalopathy [7].

DANGERS OF PROTEIN CALORIE MALNUTRITION IN LIVER DISEASE

Few, if any, controlled clinical trials have been performed to show that medical and surgical patients with protein calorie malnutrition have an increased morbidity or mortality when compared with a similar group of well nourished patients. Nevertheless, as mentioned earlier, protein calorie malnutrition is associated with impairment of immunological defence mechanisms [8], and wound healing is impaired in malnourished animals [9]. Moreover, there are studies available to show that preoperative nutritional support significantly decreases the incidence of post-operative infection [10, 11]. Taken together these findings do suggest that at least the malnourished surgical patient is at a greater risk of developing post-operative complications than a comparable well nourished patient, and there seems little reason at present to exclude malnourished patients with chronic liver disease from this category. Patients with advanced chronic parenchymal liver disease are known to have an increased susceptibility toward developing infections [12].

It is probable that the impaired host defences to infection develop not only on account of the underlying liver disease [13–15] but also on account of a potentially reversible component related to malnutrition [1]. Infection and wound breakdown are both important precipitating causes of hepatic encephalopathy in these patients. While it may not be possible to reverse the underlying hepatic pathology, improvement of the nutritional status of these patients may prove in the future to have a beneficial effect on outcome.

NUTRITIONAL SUPPORT IN THE ABSENCE OF HEPATIC ENCEPHALOPATHY

When there is no impairment of mental function, the nutritional status of malnourished patients with parenchymal liver disease can be improved by standard means. Whenever possible, this should be done by increasing normal dietary intake with appropriate supplementation with electrolytes, vitamins and haematinics. If for any reason nutrients cannot be administered in the form of a normal diet, then these patients should receive nutritional support via the enteral or parenteral route. The normal principles for determining whether nutritional support should be provided by the enteral or parenteral route should be adhered to and, in general, as long as gastrointestinal function is normal or near normal, attempts should be made to provide nutritional support via the enteral route and the use of parenteral nutrition should be restricted to those patients in whom there is severe impairment of gastrointestinal function.

NUTRITIONAL SUPPORT IN THE PRESENCE OF HEPATIC ENCEPHALOPATHY

Although the pathogenesis of hepatic encephalopathy has not been fully elucidated, for many years high blood levels of ammonia have been thought to play a major role and accordingly the rationale of standard 'anti-coma' therapy has been to lower blood ammonia levels. A major source of ammonia formation is colonic bacterial ureolysis and the cornerstone of therapy, namely protein restriction, has been aimed at reducing the rate of urea synthesis—therapy with neomycin and lactulose being aimed at further reducing colonic production and absorption of ammonia respectively.

In practice therefore many comatosed patients receive peripheral infusion of 10% dextrose as their sole source of energy and a maximum of 20 g protein via a nasogastric tube as their sole source of nitrogen. Vitamin supplementations usually being administered in the form of daily Parenterovite injections. If the patient has ascites, volume intake is restricted to 1.0–1.5 litres/day, so that total energy intake may be as low as 400 kcals/day.

The net result of this standard approach is that it has not only been impossible to improve the nutritional status of the malnourished and encephalopathic cirrhotic patients, but as implied above, the nutritional status of these patients is actually worsened during treatment.

Important advances have recently been made in our understanding of the pathogenesis of hepatic encephalopathy, particularly in relationship to imbalances in plasma amino acid profiles and brain false neurotransmitter synthesis. Based on this work, new approaches to the therapy of malnutrition in encephalopathic cirrhotic patients have been developed in which the aim is to achieve positive nitrogen balance and improvement of nutritional status, at the same time as preventing the worsening of neuropsychiatric status. There is even a suggestion in some of the recent studies that hepatic encephalopathy can actually be improved by these novel approaches to treatment.

INNOVATIVE APPROACHES TO THE NUTRITIONAL THERAPY OF ENCEPHALOPATHIC CIRRHOTIC PATIENTS

The first attempt to improve the nutritional status of encephalopathic patients with chronic parenchymal liver disease involved the parenteral administration of standard nitrogen-containing solutions. In one study, protein hydrolysate solutions were administered intravenously to 11 cirrhotic patients; positive nitrogen balance was not achieved and ammonia levels rose in all subjects [16]. Later Fischer and colleagues showed that infusion of more than 45–50 g of protein per day produced marked hepatic encephalopathy in cirrhotic patients so treated [17].

In an important series of studies, Fischer and his colleagues showed that encephalopathic cirrhotic patients exhibit imbalances of amino acid metabolism manifested by elevated plasma levels of the aromatic amino acids, phenylalanine, and tyrosine and depressed levels of the branch chain amino acids, leucine, isoleucine and valine [18–21]. These observations have been confirmed in cirrhotic patients by Sherlock and colleagues [22] and in patients with fulminant hepatic failure [23]. These changes have recently been directly implicated in the pathogenesis of hepatic encephalopathy.

The aromatic and branched-chain amino acids share a group-specific transport system on the capillary side of the blood–brain barrier. In the presence of low circulating levels of the branched chain amino acids and high levels of the aromatic amino acids, brain uptake of the latter would be expected to be increased and this has been confirmed experimentally in an experimental model of chronic liver disease [18, 24]. The resultant increased brain levels of these acids is thought to lead to alteration in brain neurotransmitter synthesis with encephalopathy developing on account of increased synthesis of the inhibitory neurotransmitters, octopamine and beta hydroxyphenylethanolamine [18–23].

Impressed with the consistency of the plasma amino acid abnormalities in cirrhotic patients with hepatic encephalopathy, Fischer and colleagues devised a specially formulated amino acid solution for intravenous use containing markedly decreased amounts of phenylalanine, tryptophan, methionine and glycine and increased amounts of the branch-chain amino acids, leucine, isoleucine and valine. After showing that survival in encephalopathic dogs receiving this formulation was significantly increased compared to dogs receiving a standard intravenous formulation of amino acids [25], clinical studies were commenced.

Results were encouraging for not only did infusion of the amino acid mixture correct plasma amino acid profiles of patients, but positive nitrogen balance was achieved [20]. Moreover, there appeared to be an improvement rather than deterioration in mental state during treatment.

These findings therefore suggested that a parenteral amino acid solution with a pattern complementing the abnormal plasma amino acid profiles seen in encephalopathic patients could prove beneficial, not only in preventing a deterioration in nutritional status but also in improving the mental status of these patients.

Since the publication of Fischer's data, a good deal of controversy has arisen as to the efficacy of the various branched-chain amino acid enriched diets. The problem has been compounded by the fact that different regimes have been administered to different groups of patients. For example, branched-chain amino acids have been administered enterally and parenterally, in the presence or absence of additional amino acid sources of nitrogen, as well as varying amounts of dietary protein. The various diets have been administered to cirrhotic patients with overt and latent encephalopathy. Moreover, those patients with overt encephalopathy who have received these diets have both acute mental deterioration as well as established chronic encephalopathy usually developing, for example, following previous portacaval decompression for bleeding oesophageal varices.

Although it is therefore not easy to dissect out hard evidence in favour or against the use of the various regimes, results of several controlled studies are now becoming available. One of the most important of these shows that branched-chain amino acids, when administered parenterally as the sole source of nitrogen to cirrhotic patients with acute encephalopathy, had no significantly beneficial effect upon clinical or EEG signs of encephalopathy, as compared with complete nitrogen restriction and, indeed, there was a strong suggestion that mortality was greater in the treatment rather than control group [26]. There are few other controlled studies available that have tested the efficacy of branched-chain amino acid enriched diets in cirrhotic patients with acute hepatic encephalopathy. However, the above study argues strongly against the use of branched-chain amino acid diets as the sole source of nitrogen, and diets used in future studies will almost certainly contain other essential amino acids.

With regard to the effect that dietary supplementation with branched-chain amino acids have on the mental state of chronically encephalopathic cirrhotic patients, no beneficial effect was seen in one carefully controlled cross-over study [27]. Significant improvements were seen in formal psychometric tests performed on cirrhotic patients without clinically evident encephalopathy in a further study [28], although it is unlikely that the changes found would be clinically significant. It would seem therefore that in respect of chronically encephalopathic patients dietary supplementation with branched chain amino acids is not likely to substantially improve the mental status of these patients.

The preliminary results of an American co-operative controlled trial have recently been published [29]. Patients with established chronic hepatic encephalopathy were randomised to receive a specifically formulated elemental diet where the free amino acid nitrogen source has been designed to complement the plasma amino acid changes (Hepaticaid) or standard dietary protein restriction. No significant improvements occurred in the treatment group with respect to coma grading, but the nutritional status of the patients was improved.

It seems likely, therefore, that the main role of these specially formulated diets will be directed towards improving the nutritional rather than mental status of encephalopathic cirrhotic patients. It should be stressed, though, that a good deal of the evidence available at present does suggest that it is possible to increase dietary nitrogen intake in those patients using the specially formulated branched chain enriched diets without detriment to the mental status. This in itself, if confirmed by future studies, will still represent a significant advance in relationship to patient management.

On the basis of the results that are available to date, we recommend the use of the specially formulated nutritional products available for enteral and parenteral administration as a means of either improving or preventing further deterioration in the nutritional status of malnourished encephalopathic patients, rather than as a primary means of improving mental status. Both the parenteral and enteral diets used in our Unit have as their nitrogen source a mixture of free L-amino acids, the formulation of which differs from standard parenteral and enteral diets in that the proportion of branched chain amino acids is increased and the aromatics and methionine reduced. It should be noted that neither diet contains tyrosine or cystine. A recent study indicates that it may prove difficult to place some patients in positive nitrogen balance with these diets until supplements of these two amino acids are provided [30].

PARENTERAL NUTRITION REGIMES

Table 9.1 shows the composition of a specially formulated infusion solution, one litre of which contains 40 g amino acids, equivalent to 6.25 g nitrogen. The principle difference between this solution and most standard amino acid solutions is the markedly decreased levels of phenylalanine, methionine and tryptophan. The concentrations of the branched chain amino acids are increased. Glucose constitutes the energy source and the non-protein energy to nitrogen ratio is 193:1. The sodium content is low and the solution is potassium-free.

Technique of administration

A full clinical, biochemical and immunological assessment

Table 9.1 Composition of the parenteral infusion solution in a volume of one litre.

Amino acid composition	grams/litre
L-leucine	5.5
L-isoleucine	4.5
L-glycine	4.5
L-lysine	3.8
L-valine	4.2
L-proline	4.0
L-alanine	3.75
L-arginine	3.0
L-serine	2.5
L-threonine	2.25
L-histidine	1.20
L-methionine	0.5
L-phenylalanine	0.5
L-tryptophan	0.38
L-cysteine	0.2
Total protein as amino acids	40.0 g
Total nitrogen	6.25 g
Glucose 230 g	920 cals
HCl/litre	40 mmol
Na acetate/litre	30 mmol
$MgSO_4$/litre	4 mmol
Phosphate	12.5 mmol
Calcium	2 mmol

should be made of nutritional status and encephalopathy graded clinically (Table 9.2) before treatment is instituted. An EEG should be performed prior to treatment and, if physically and neurologically possible, a Reitan trail test performed [31].

The infusion solution should be administered through a silicone catheter positioned in the left subclavian vein and, because patients with chronic parenchymal liver disease already have an increased susceptibility toward developing infection, meticulous care must be taken in managing the catheter entry site.

Infusions of the solution should begin at the rate of 1 litre per day (Table 9.3) for the first 24 hours (6.25 g nitrogen, 920 non-protein calories/day). The dose can then be increased by 0.5 litres/day up to a maximum of 2 litres/day (12.5 g nitrogen, 1840 non-protein calories) providing the patients' neuropsychiatric status does not deteriorate, and electrolyte disturbances do not occur. Infusion will have to be restricted to 1.5–2.0 litres/day if ascites is present. In other patients the dose may be increased above 2 litres if clinical conditions permit.

Supplementation with minerals, potassium and vitamins will often be required (Table 9.3) and other supplements may have to be added to the regime, depending on the biochemical status of the patient.

Patient monitoring

The principles involved in patient monitoring are the same as

Table 9.2 Clinical stages in development of hepatic coma.

Grade	Mental state
I	Euphoria, occasionally depression Fluctuant, mild confusion Sluggish thinking Untidy. Slurred speech Disorder in sleep rhythm
II	Accentuation of I. Drowsy Inappropriate behaviour
III	Sleeps most of the time but is rousable Incoherent speech. Marked confusion
IV	Unrousable. May or may not respond to noxious stimuli

Table 9.3 Parenteral nutrition regime for patients with chronic parenchymal liver disease with hepatic encephalopathy.

Day	Volume (litres)	Nitrogen content (grams)	Non-protein energy (kcal)	Sodium (mmol)
1	1.0	6.25	920	30
2	1.5	9.38	1380	45
3	2.0	12.5	1840	60

Supplements (all daily)

	Additive	Route of administration
Minerals	Addamel 10 ml	Add to infusion
Potassium	KCl solution BP (1.5 mg/10 ml) 2 vials K^+ and Cl^- 40 mmol	Add to infusion
Vitamins	Parenterovite vials 1 & 2	Add to infusion
	Vitamin K 10 mg*	i.m.

* Indicated if prothrombin time is prolonged

those involved in the monitoring of any patient receiving parenteral nutrition; as many of the patients will often have severe underlying biochemical abnormalities, particular care must be taken to ensure that electrolyte, calcium, magnesium, zinc and phosphate levels remain within normal limits.

Careful monitoring of neuropsychiatric status should also be performed. Daily clinical grading is necessary, and if patients are physically and neurologically capable, daily Reitan trail tests should also be performed. Electroencephalograms should be performed daily for the first 3 days of treatment and thereafter at frequent intervals.

The infusion rate should be cut back by half a litre a day (a reduction of 3.13 g nitrogen) if there is a deterioration in one grade of coma in the absence of a demonstrable precipitating cause. Infusion should be stopped altogether if there is a more rapid deterioration in neuropsychiatric status.

Other standard therapy for hepatic encephalopathy (neomycin, lactulose, daily or twice-daily magnesium sulphate enemata) should be continued throughout parenteral nutrition. If there is a marked and sustained improvement in mental state then these can be discontinued.

ENTERAL NUTRITION

Of the 148 patients who have received enteral nutrition in our unit during the last year, 30% were unconscious when treatment was instituted. In the light of this, we have felt confident that nutritional support can be provided to encephalopathic cirrhotic patients via the enteral route. As the administration of large quantities of whole protein has a deleterious effect upon neuropsychiatric status of these patients, none of the currently available polymeric enteric feeds (Clinifeed, Triosorbon, Isocal, Ensure) can be safely administered. Similarly, the two elemental diets (Vivonex, Flexical) whose nitrogen sources are based upon the amino acid composition of whole protein, are equally unsuitable. A new elemental diet has been developed in America whose nitrogen source has been specially formulated according to the amino acid composition of the parenteral nutrition solution. This diet, marketed under the name Hepaticaid (Boots) is currently being used in our unit and at the Royal Free Hospital and will soon become more widely available in the UK.

The composition of the diet is shown in Table 9.4. The nitrogen

Table 9.4 Composition of Hepaticaid*.

Amino acid composition (g/package)			
L-leucine	2.008	L-phenylalanine	0.180
L-isoleucine	1.643	L-tryptophan	0.120
Glycine	1.643		
L-lysine acetate	1.575	Total protein as	
(free base)	1.116	amino acids	14.5 g
L-valine	1.533	Total nitrogen	2.23 g
L-proline	1.460	Carbohydrate	97.7 g
L-alanine	1.397	Fat	12.3 g
L-arginine	1.095	Total calories	560
L-serine	0.912		
L-threonine	0.820	Non-protein	
L-histidine	0.438	energy/nitrogen	
L-methionine	0.182	ratio	224:1

* Unlike the standard proprietary enteric diets, Hepaticaid is not a nutritionally complete diet and does not contain electrolytes, minerals, trace elements or vitamins

source is composed of L-amino acids and contains relatively large proportions of the branched-chain amino acids, small amounts of phenylalanine and no tyrosine at all. The energy source consists predominantly of medium chain length glucose polymers with smaller quantities of triglycerides.

Technique of administration

In the technique of administration used in our unit, a full clinical, biochemical and immunological assessment is made of nutritional status, and encephalopathy graded according to standard clinical criteria (Table 9.2) before treatment is commenced. In addition, an EEG is performed prior to treatment, and the Reitan trail test carried out in patients with grades I–II encephalopathy.

We administer Hepaticaid by pump-assisted constant gravity infusion via a one millimetre internal diameter feeding tube positioned in the stomach. To date we have not shown the presence of oesophageal varices to be a contraindication to nasogastric feeding.

Our aim is to use Hepaticaid as the sole source of nutrition in these patients, and treatment is prescribed for 7–10 days, depending on the clinical status of the patient, before a normal diet is gradually reintroduced. Each package of Hepaticaid contains approx. 2.23 g nitrogen and 560 calories (Table 9.4) and our standard regime (Table 9.5) is based upon increasing increments of these values. When ascites is present, fluid restriction to 1.5 litres/day is often necessary.

By virtue of its free amino acid nitrogen source, the osmolality of Hepaticaid is high, and if there are no clinical indications for fluid restriction, the final volume can be increased up to 2–3 litres/day.

Hepaticaid is electrolyte-free and does not contain minerals, trace elements or vitamins. Supplements of these are therefore routinely administered (Table 9.5).

As mentioned above, treatment is usually continued for 7–10 days. If the mental state of the patient has improved by this time, we gradually reintroduce a normal diet. Patients are started on a 20 g protein intake, which is increased by 20 g daily increments at the same time as the intake of Hepaticaid is reduced by 1 package a day (2.23 g nitrogen, 14.5 g protein as amino acids). The final daily dietary protein intake will be determined by the clinical and mental state of the patient.

Patient monitoring

Because Hepaticaid is not a nutritionally complete diet, we take

Table 9.5   Enteral nutrition regime.

Day	Grams nitrogen/day	Calories	Non-protein energy to nitrogen ratio (kCal/g N)	Final total vol. (ml)
1	4.5	1120	224:1	1000
2	6.7	1680	224:1	1000
3	8.9	2240	224:1	1500
4	11.2	2800	224:1	1500

Supplements (all daily)

Supplement	Additive	Route of administration
Minerals	Addamel 10 ml	Add to diet
Potassium	KCl solution BP (1.5 mg/10 ml) 2-vials K^+ and Cl^- 40 mmol	Add to diet
Vitamins	Parenterovite vials 1 & 2	i.v.
	Thiamine 200 mg t.d.s.	Orally or add to diet
	Folic acid 5 mg t.d.s.	Orally or add to diet
	Vitamin K 10 mg*	i.m.

* Indicated if prothrombin time prolonged

particular care to ensure that electrolyte, calcium, magnesium, zinc and phosphate levels remain within normal limits.

The neuropsychiatric status of our patients is monitored closely. We would recommend that daily clinical grading (Table 9.2) is necessary, and if patients are physically and neurologically able to do so, daily Reitan trail tests should also be performed. We perform electroencephalograms before treatment is commenced and at frequent intervals thereafter. If there is a deterioration of 1 coma grade in the absence of a demonstrable precipitating cause (gastrointestinal haemorrhage, electrolyte disturbances, sepsis, etc.) we reduce intake of the diet by 1 packet per day (2.23 g nitrogen), and intake of the diet is discontinued if there is a more rapid deterioration in neuropsychiatric status.

As with the parenteral nutrition regimes, standard therapy for hepatic encephalopathy (neomycin, lactulose and bowel enemata) is continued during enteral nutrition and discontinued only when there is a marked and sustained improvement in mental state.

To date we have administered the diet to 10 malnourished cirrhotic patients (aged 35–72 years) admitted in grades I–III hepatic coma. The 10 patients received Hepaticaid for between 3 and 23 days (mean 7.3 days). Positive nitrogen balance was achieved by day 3 and maintained in all patients fed for 7 days or more, and no problems were encountered with the use of either the diet or the fine bore tubes in these patients.

The mental state of 8 of the 10 patients improved markedly during the treatment period until encephalopathy could not be clinically detected (Fig. 9.1). One patient, however, deteriorated to grade IV coma and died in hepatorenal failure and one patient, after an initial improvement in mental state was noted, reverted to grade II coma at the time of receiving an inadvertent Heminevrin infusion.

Serial plasma amino acid changes were monitored throughout the study, and while plasma levels of methionine and phenylalanine remained unchanged, tyrosine levels fell significantly ($p < 0.05$), branched chain levels rose ($p < 0.05$) resulting in a significant elevation of the branched chain to aromatic amino acid ratio ($p < 0.01$). Plasma ammonia levels, elevated at the start of the study, remained unchanged despite improvement in amino acid profile and mental state of the patients.

Our experience using this specially formulated enteral diet therefore suggests that it is possible to safely increase nitrogen intake in malnourished encephalopathic patients with acute encephalopathy without worsening hepatic encephalopathy. The study was uncontrolled, however, so the data do not imply a beneficial effect on outcome and no conclusions can be drawn in respect of possible primary therapeutic effect on hepatic encephalopathy.

MALNUTRITION IN FULMINANT HEPATIC FAILURE

Fulminant hepatic failure is by definition the clinical syndrome that occurs as a result of massive hepatic necrosis of liver cells in a patient who has had no previous evidence of liver disease [32]. It is characterised by the onset of a severe progressive encephalopathy and its mortality rate, which is closely related to the severity of the encephalopathy, is as high as 80–90% in those who develop signs of grade IV coma [33]. The usual causes of fulminant hepatic failure are viral hepatitis, paracetamol overdose, halothane and other drug hypersensitivities. The condition is notable because the natural history of the disease is often very short and accordingly malnutrition usually develops in survivors on account of therapeutic regimes rather than longstanding impaired intake of nutrients.

It has recently become clear that no unified concept is ever likely to explain adequately the pathogenesis of the acute hepatic encephalopathy that characterises fulminant hepatic failure [34]. Persuasive experimental evidence favours a contributory role for the raised plasma levels of many low-molecular weight toxins existing in the circulation both as the water soluble native form, e.g. ammonium and amino acids, and bound to plasma proteins (such as phenolic acid, fatty acids, bile acids and bilirubin). In addition, Opolon and colleagues [35] provided evidence that compounds in the middle-molecular weight range of 1500–5000 were also likely to be important. Successful reversal of coma in acute liver failure thus requires a means of support capable of removing this wide range of potentially toxic compounds.

To date, a number of artificial liver support systems have been developed and used in the clinical setting. Of these, the most encouraging results have been obtained using polyacrylonitrile haemodialysis [36, 37]. A notable feature of this and other support systems, such as charcoal haemoperfusion, has been the removal of large quantities of amino acids from the circulation of the treated patients [36]. Unquestionably, this contributes in a major way to the protein malnutrition that is evident in survivors who regain consciousness.

Patients with fulminant hepatic failure who recover do so completely, quite unlike those with underlying chronic liver disease. This is due to the considerable regenerative capacity of the liver. When consciousness is regained, efforts should be made to improve the nutritional status of these patients. In the light of our recent knowledge about the use of specially formulated parenteral and enteral nutritional regimes, it seems reasonable to expect that survivors should be treated with one or either of these following artificial liver support and before receiving a normal diet.

REFERENCES

1 O'Keefe S.J., Carraher T.G., El-Zayadi A.R., *et al* (1980) Malnutrition and immuno-incompetence in patients with liver disease. *Lancet* ii, 615.
2 Mezey E.M. (1978) Liver disease and nutrition. *Gastroenterology* 74, 770.
3 Leevy C.M., Baker H., Tentlove W., *et al* (1965) B-complex vitamins in liver disease in the alcoholic. *Am. J. Clin. Nutr.* 16, 339.
4 Mezey E. & Faillace L.A. (1971) Metabolic impairment and recovery time in acute ethanol intoxication. *J. Nerv. Ment. Dis.* 153, 445.
5 Van Goidsenhoven G.E., Henke W.J., Vacca J.B., *et al* (1963) Pancreatic function in cirrhosis of the liver. *Am. J. Dig. Dis.* 8, 160.

6   Mezey E. (1975) Intestinal function in chronic alcoholism. *Ann. NY Acad. Sci.* **252**, 215.

7   Jones E.A., Sherlock S. & Crowley N. (1967) Bacteraemia in association with hepatocellular and hepatobiliary disease. *Postgrad. Med. J.* Suppl 43, 7.

8   Alexander J.W. (1974) Emerging concepts in the control of surgical infections. *Surgery* **75**, 934.

9   Scrimshaw N.S., Taylor C.E. & Gordon J.E. (1968) Interactions of nutrition in infection. *WHO monograph No. 57.* World Health Organisation, Geneva.

10   Bojanowicz K. (1977) Anwendung der chemisch definierten Diat bei und nach Kolonkarzinom operationen. *Z. Ernaehrungswissenschaft* Suppl 20, 14.

11   Heatley R.V., Williams R.H.P. & Lewis M.H. (1979) Pre-operative intravenous feeding—a controlled trial. *Postgrad. Med. J.* **55**, 541.

12   Faulk W.P., Demaeyer E.M. & Davies A.J.S. (1974) Some effects of malnutrition on the immune responses in man. *Am. J. Clin. Nutr.* **27**, 638.

13   Fox R.H., Dudley F.J., Samuels M., *et al.* (1973) Lymphocyte transformation in response to phytohaemagglutinin in primary biliary cirrhosis. The search for a plasma inhibiting factor. *Gut* **89**, 89.

14   Hsu C.L.S. & Leary C.M. (1971) Inhibition of PHA-stimulated lymphocyte transformation by plasma from patients with advanced alcoholic cirrhosis. *Clin. Exp. Immunol.* **8**, 749.

15   Van Epps D.E., Stickland R.G. & Williams R.C. (1975) Inhibitions of leucocyte chemotaxis in alcoholic liver disease. *Am. J. Med.* **59**, 200.

16   Host W.R., Serlin O. & Rush B.F. (1972) Hyperalimentation in cirrhotic patients. *Am. J. Surg.* **123**, 57.

17   Fischer J.E., Yoshimura N., Aguirre A., James J.H., Cummings M.G., Abel R.M. & Deindoerfer F. (1974) Plasma amino acids in patients with hepatic encephalopathy. *Am. J. Surg.* **127**, 40.

18   James J.H., Escourrou J. & Fischer J.E. (1978) Blood brain neutral amino acid transport activity is increased after portocaval anastomosis. *Science* **200**, 1395.

19   James J.H., Ziparo V., Jeppsson B., *et al* (1979) Hyperammonaemia, plasma amino acid imbalance and blood brain amino acid transport: a united theory of portal-systemic encephalopathy. *Lancet* **ii**, 772.

20   Fischer J.E., Rosen H.M., Ebeid A.M., *et al* (1976) The effect of normalisation of plasma amino acids on hepatic encephalopathy in man. *Surgery* **80**, 77.

21   Rosen H.M., Yoshimura N., Hodgman S.M., *et al* (1977) Plasma amino acid patterns in hepatic encephalopathy of differing etiology. *Gastroenterology* **72**, 483.

22   Morgan M.Y., Milson J.P. & Sherlock S. (1978) Plasma ratio of valine, leucine and isoleucine to phenylalanine and tyrosine in liver disease. *Gut* **19**, 1068.

23   Chase R.A., Davis M., Trewby P.M., *et al* (1978) Plasma amino acid profiles in patients with fulminant hepatic failure treated by repeated polyacrylonitrile hemodialysis. *Gastroenterology* **75**, 1033.

24 Zaki A., Williams R. & Silk D.B.A. (1980) Increases in blood brain barrier permeability after portocaval anastomosis. *Gut* **21**, A900.

25 Fischer J.E., Funovics J.M., Aguirre A., *et al* (1975) The role of plasma amino acids in hepatic encephalopathy. *Surgery* **78**, 276.

26 Wahren J., Denis J., Desurmont P., *et al* (1981) Is i.v. administration of BCAA effective in the treatment of hepatic encephalopathy—A multicentre study. In *Proceedings 3rd European Congress on Parenteral and Enteral Nutrition*, 61.

27 Eriksson S., Persson A. & Wahren J. (1981) Failure of oral branched chain amino acids to improve chronic hepatic encephalopathy. In *Proceedings 3rd European Congress on Parenteral and Enteral Nutrition* 62.

28 Holm E., Langhans E., Meisinger L., *et al* (1981) BCAA-enriched diets for oral treatment of patients with liver cirrhosis: A controlled study of biochemical variables, psychometric performance and the EEG. In *Proceedings 3rd European Congress on Parenteral and Enteral Nutrition* p. 59.

29 Horse D., Grace N., Conn H.O., *et al* (1981) A double blind randomized comparison of dietary protein and anoral branched chain amino acid (BCAA) supplement in cirrhotic patients with chronic portal-systemic encephalopathy (PSE). *Hepatology* **1**,518.

30 Rudman D., Kutner M., Ansley J., *et al* (1981) Hypotyrosinemia, hypocystinemia and failure to retain nitrogen during total parenteral nutrition of cirrhotic patients. *Gastroenterology* **81**, 1025.

31 Zeegan R., Drinkwater J.E. & Dawson A.M. (1970) Method for measuring cerebral dysfunction in patients with liver disease. *Br. Med. J.* **2**, 633.

32 Trey C. & Davidson C.S. (1980) The management of fulminant hepatic failure. In *Progress in Liver Disease* 3, eds. H. Popper and F. Schaffner, p. 282. Grune and Stratton, New York.

33 Silk D.B.A. & Williams R. (1978) Experiences in the treatment of fulminant hepatic failure by conservative therapy, charcoal haemoperfusion, and polyacrylonitrile haemodialysis. *Int. J. Artif. Organs* **1**, 29.

34 Silk D.B.A. & Williams R. (1979) Acute liver failure. *Br. J. Hosp. Med.* **22**, 437.

35 Opolon P., Lavallard M.C., Huguet C., *et al* (1976) Haemodialysis versus gross haemodialysis in experimental hepatic coma. *Surg. Gynaecol. Obstet.* **142**, 845.

36 Silk D.B.A., Trewby P.N., Chase R.A., *et al* (1977) Treatment of fulminant hepatic failure by polycarylonitrile membrane haemodialysis. *Lancet* **ii**, 1.

37 Denis J., Opolon P., Nusinovici V., *et al* (1978) Treatment of encephalopathy during fulminant hepatic failure with high permeability membrane. *Gut* **19**, 787.

Chapter 10
The Kidney and Nutrition

This chapter is restricted to the nutritional management of patients with established chronic renal failure and those developing acute renal failure, both of whom become malnourished as a result of co-existing medical or surgical problems. The nutritional management of the stable out-patient with chronic renal failure is not considered.

It should be appreciated from the outset that catabolic patients with renal failure, from a metabolic point of view, behave in a similar way to normal patients with respect to their response to injury and sepsis [1]. It is the catabolism of body protein (often as high as 100–120 g/day) that has such a deleterious effect in renal failure, for it is the concomitant release of potentially toxic intra-cellular substances into the extracellular space that forms the basis of the uraemic syndrome. The overall aim of nutritional support in injured patients with renal failure is therefore to provide a sufficient number of calories and nitrogen to reverse the gluconeogenic response to injury and prevent the release of toxic substances into the circulation [2, 3].

The importance of improving or reversing negative nitrogen balance in malnourished renal patients cannot be overstated. It is the associated impaired humoral and cellular immunocompetence that predisposes these patients to infection and, as has been well documented, infection is a common cause of mortality in those patients in whom acute renal failure has developed as a complication of pre-existing underlying disease processes [4].

ACUTE RENAL FAILURE

In patients with acute renal failure complicating surgery or severe trauma, the mortality is about 60%, with mortality in medical acute renal failure cases being around 45% [1, 4]. The principles involved in the nutritional management of patients with acute renal failure are governed by a number of important principles (see Table 10.1).

Table 10.1 Important factors governing the nutritional management of patients with acute renal failure.

1 Degree of catabolism—principles governed by nitrogen losses
2 Severity of the renal failure—requirements for dialysis
3 Function of gastrointestinal tract—enteral or parenteral support
4 Extra renal losses—extra fluid and electrolyte requirements (e.g. fistulae, gastric aspirates)

Degree of catabolism

Careful monitoring of nitrogen balance is essential in these patients so that the degree of catabolism can be estimated. This is so because the principles of nutritional support are governed by nitrogen losses. Thus, the patients with a modest degree of catabolism can be managed conservatively by a high energy, low protein regime, whereas there is quite definitely no place for protein restriction in the more catabolic patients. Standard principles of nutritional support have to be adhered to in these patients and they will require frequent dialysis to accommodate nutritional fluid volumes.

Calculation of nitrogen losses [2]

It is important to carefully estimate the nitrogen losses of the malnourished renal failure patient. This can usually be performed by using the simple formulae for computing nitrogen losses from urinary urea excretion values (see Chapter 4). However, corrections have to be made when the blood urea (BU) is rising and if there is proteinuria.

$$\text{Nitrogen loss (g/24 hours)} = \text{mmol urinary urea/24 hours} \times 0.028 + 2 = A$$

$$\text{Nitrogen loss as proteinuria (g/24 hours)} = \frac{\text{g protein/24 hours}}{6.25} = B$$

Nitrogen loss as rising blood urea (g/24 hours)

$$(\text{Rise in BU (mmol/l)}) \times \frac{60}{100}(\text{kg body wt}) \times 0.028 = C$$

Total nitrogen losses g/24 hours $= A + B + C$

Requirements for dialysis

Catabolic patients with acute renal failure require frequent dialysis. The provision of nutritional support does not reduce dialysis requirements and indeed, due to the need to accommodate administered fluids, dialysis requirements usually increase. Haemodialysis rather than peritoneal dialysis is the method of choice because losses of whole protein and amino acids are less. As Table 10.2 shows, protein losses in a daily 40 litre peritoneal dialysis may vary between 20 and 40 g, with 13–15 g of amino acids lost. On the other hand during haemodialysis no whole protein is lost (most standard dialysis membranes are permeable to compounds with a molecular weight of up to 200 daltons) and losses of amino acids usually lie in the range of 2–3 g/hour.

In the light of the above comments, it follows that catabolic patients are best managed in specialist units with haemodialysis facilities. For obvious reasons referral to such units should be considered early rather than late.

Gastrointestinal function

As with non-uraemic patients, decisions have to be made as to whether to provide nutritional support via the enteral or parenteral routes. In the author's experience, a significant number of modestly catabolic patients with acute renal failure have normal gastrointestinal function and can be fed enterally. On the other hand many catabolic patients with acute renal failure have impaired gastrointestinal function and have to be fed parenterally.

Extrarenal losses

In the patients we see with acute renal failure, renal failure has developed as a late complication of other serious underlying disorders. It is most common, for example, for renal failure to develop in patients being nursed in our intensive care unit rather than the general hospital wards. Consequently, we have found that these patients have complicated metabolic and electrolyte disturbances, and are often losing fluid and electrolytes from gastrointestinal fistulae, in high volume gastric aspirates or in

Table 10.2 Nitrogen losses during dialysis. (After [2])

Type of dialysis procedure	Protein losses (g/day)	Amino acid losses (g/day)
Peritoneal (40 litres/day)	20–30	13–15
Haemodialysis (3 hour/day)	None	6–9

high output drain effluents. Proper care of these patients must
involve close monitoring of these losses, together with careful
analysis of their electrolyte and nitrogen content.

169
*The Kidney
and Nutrition*

NUTRITIONAL MANAGEMENT

Approaches to nutritional management differ according to the
nitrogen losses, or degree of catabolism (see Table 10.3).

Modest catabolism (nitrogen loss 10–14 g/day)

As mentioned above, patients with a modest rise of blood urea of
4–6 mmol/day and nitrogen losses of 10–14 g nitrogen/day can
be managed conservatively by the enteral or parenteral route
with a protein restriction regime (0.3 g/kg body weight per day of
protein and 40–50 kcal/kg body weight per day). With respect to
fluid requirements the time honoured approach of 500 ml/day of
fluid plus any fluid losses from the previous day, e.g. urine,
diarrhoea, fistula and other losses from the gastrointestinal tract,
remains appropriate. The electrolyte content of such regimes will
have to be modified with respect to sodium (20–30 mmol/day)
and potassium (below 40 mmol/day) content. As with other
patients careful checks should be kept on calcium, phosphate and
magnesium requirements and adequate vitamin, mineral and
essential element supplements should be given.

When these patients require dialysis it is important to make
allowances for the extra losses incurred (Table 10.2). In peritoneal dialysis, substantial losses of protein and amino acids

Table 10.3 Nutritional management of patients with acute renal failure
(After [2])

Groups	Rise in blood urea mmol/day	Nitrogen losses g/day	Principles of nutritional management
Modest catabolism	4–6	10–14	Protein restriction (0.3 g protein/kg) High energy (45–50 kcal/kg)
Moderately high catabolism	6–10	14–24	Satisfy all nutritional requirements.
Severe catabolism	10–12	24–29	Dialyse frequently

occur, whereas with haemodialysis only amino acids are lost. A number of recent studies have shown that amino acid losses during dialysis procedures can be minimised by adding free amino acids to the dialysis fluid (70–90 mg/litre), equivalent to 10 ml Synthamin 9/litre dialysis fluid [2].

As with other malnourished patients, nutrients should be provided by the enteral route whenever possible. Parenteral nutrition should be resorted to *only* if enteral nutrition is not feasible.

Enteral feeding of patients with modest nitrogen losses

The relatively high sodium and potassium content of the standard whole-protein-containing enteric feeds prohibits their use in the majority of modestly catabolic patients in renal failure. Our enteral feeding regime is based upon the use of a diet whose nitrogen source consists of essential free amino acids and energy source of a mixture of glucose polymers and triglycerides (Amin-Aid; Boots, Nottingham). We do not believe that it is of crucial importance to use only essential amino acids, and other similarly constituted diets with low sodium and potassium levels and containing a wider range of amino acids would be equally suitable.

Suggested regimes are shown in Table 10.4. AminAid contains no vitamins, haematinics or essential biological elements, so supplementation of the feeding regimes will be required. The additives and suggested sources are shown in Table 10.5. All can be added directly to the diets during stirring or blending as long as the tablets are crushed to a powder beforehand.

Table 10.4 Enteral feeding regime in modestly catabolic patients with acute renal failure.

Volume	Packets of AminAid*	Grams of nitrogen (amino acid g)	Energy (kcal) Carbo-hydrate	Fat	Total	Na^+ (mmol)	K^+
1020	3	3.2 (19.8)	1320	648	1968	6	6
1360	4	4.2 (26.4)	1760	864	2624	8	8
1700	5	5.3 (33.0)	2200	1080	3280	10	10

All regimes will require supplementation with vitamins, haematinics and essential biological elements. All may need additions of phosphorus, potassium, magnesium and zinc depending on circulating levels (see Table 10.5)
* Each packet added slowly to 250 ml boiled water and stirred or blended. Final volume is approximately 340 ml

Table 10.5. Additives for enteral feeding regimes in renal failure.

Additive	Suggested sources
Water soluble vitamins	1 vial of Solvito daily
Fat soluble vitamins	1 vial Vitlipid daily
Vitamin B12	1000 μg i.m. when required
Folic acid	
Manganese	2 tablets Folicin daily
Ferrous sulphate	
Zinc	1–2 tablets Zincomed daily
Sodium	NaCl 1.8% w/v (300 mmol Na$^+$/litre)
	NaCl 300 mg tabs (5 mmol/l Na$^+$)
Potassium	KCl 1 mg/ml BP (20 mmol/l)
Calcium	Calcium gluconate
	(2.25 mmol/10 ml)

We feed patients by pump-assisted gravity infusion through a one millimetre diameter feeding tube positioned in the stomach. Very careful biochemical monitoring of the enterally fed renal failure patient is essential, so that the biochemistry can be normalised as early as possible (p. 176).

The regimes shown in Table 10.4 are based on requirements of protein in the order of 0.3 g protein/kg with energy requirements in the range of 45–50 kcal/kg. At first sight, it may seem that the fluid volume requirements of these types of regime would exclude this approach to management. However, if adequate dialysis is used sufficient fluid can be removed to accommodate daily enteral nutritional requirements.

Parenteral nutrition in modestly catabolic patients

The energy substrates used for feeding patients need not be significantly different from those used for the non-uraemic patient. The nitrogen source should consist of a free amino acid mixture rather than a partial hydrolysate of whole protein, as the peptide component of the hydrolysate may not be excreted as in normals, with the result that blood urea levels will rise.

A number of studies have clearly shown the benefits of parenteral nutrition in renal failure, particularly with respect to mortality [5, 6]. For the patient with modest catabolism, a suggested regime based on approximate requirements of 0.3 g protein/kg and an energy requirement of 45–50 kcal/kg is shown in Table 10.6, and the additives, if required, in Table 10.7. As with the enteral feeding regime it may seem that the fluid volume requirements of these types of regime would exclude this approach to management. However, if adequate dialysis is used, sufficient fluid can be removed from the patient to accommodate the daily intravenous nutritional volume requirements.

Hypercatabolic patients (nitrogen loss 14–30 g/day)

In these patients there is no place for severely restricted protein regimes. Management of these patients presents particularly difficult problems. As the uraemic syndrome develops consequent upon the accumulation of intracellular protein breakdown products, they will require frequent dialysis which, because of asso-

Table 10.6 Parenteral nutrition regimes in modestly catabolic renal failure patients.

Regime	Volume (litre)	Source*	Grams of nitrogen (amino acid g)	Carbohydrate (kcal)	Energy Fat (kcal)	Total	Na⁺ K⁺ (mMol)
A	0.5	Synthamin 9†	4.7 (27.5)				— —
	1.0	50% dextrose		2000			— —
Total	1.5					2000	
B	0.5	Synthamin 9†	4.7 (27.5)				— —
	0.5	20% intralipid			1000		— —
	0.5	50% dextrose		1000			— —
Total	1.5					2000	

* Synthamin 9 may be replaced by either Vamin–glucose or Vamin N. Both contain 25 mmol Na⁺/0.5 l and 10 mmol K⁺/0.5 l
† Electrolyte free

Table 10.7 Additives for parenteral feeding regimes in renal failure.

Additives	Suggested sources
Water soluble vitamins	1 vial Solivito daily
Fat soluble vitamins*	1 vial Vitlipid daily
Vitamin B12	1000 μg i.m. as required
Minerals and trace elements	1 vial Addamel daily
Potassium	KCl 1 mg/ml BP (20 mmol/l)
Sodium	NaCl 1.8% w/v (300 mmol Na⁺/litre)
Calcium	Calcium gluconate (2.25 mmol/10 ml)
Phosphate	Phosphate solution (Boots, UK) (Potassium 19 mmol/l, phosphate 100 mmol/l)

ciated nitrogen loss due to the dialysis procedure itself, will accentuate the negative nitrogen balance. As mentioned previously, haemodialysis is the dialysis method of choice, and there is no doubt, therefore, that such patients should be referred to specialist renal centres, and referral should be considered early rather than late.

Use of pure essential amino acid nitrogen sources

Claims have been made that there are advantages to using a mixture of essential amino acids rather than standard amino acid mixtures as the nitrogen source in parenteral nutrition regimes designed for patients with acute renal failure [6]. This concept has been based on a number of premises, namely that even small amounts of non-essential nitrogen may cause a worsening of uraemia [6], and that, based on work in obesity and chronic renal failure [7, 8], the circulating urea can be utilised as a source of nitrogen for protein synthesis, thereby obviating the inclusion of non-essential amino acids in the administered nitrogen regime.

A careful review of the literature reveals, however, a distinct lack of evidence that urea nitrogen recycling occurs in acute renal failure, and that it has to be appreciated that, even in chronic renal failure, such recycling processes at best account for 6% of protein synthetic requirements [3].

Nevertheless, the initial results of using a regime based on essential amino acids alone were encouraging, and patients receiving a mixture based on essential amino acids and dextrose faired better than those receiving hypertonic dextrose alone [5]. Thus, the dialysis requirements of the two patient groups did not differ significantly, mortality was significantly lower in the treatment group than in the control group, and blood urea levels differed significantly also, higher levels being noted in the patients receiving dextrose alone.

These patients commonly have associated gastrointestinal failure, and will commonly require parenteral, rather than enteral, nutrition. The basic philosophy is that, despite problems with fluid requirements, parenteral nutrition formulations are designed on a similar basis to those used in non-uraemic catabolic patients, with frequent haemodialysis being performed to accommodate parenteral nutritional volume requirements [2, 3]. As amino acids are lost during haemodialysis the intravenous regimes should be programmed so that amino acids are given between dialysis. A suitable way to compensate for nitrogen losses during dialysis is to give 500 ml of a standard free-amino acid solution (4.5 g nitrogen/500 ml) during 2–3 hours haemodialysis.

Table 10.8 summarises the basic constituents of the essential amino acid formulation, as used by Abel and his colleagues [5, 6]. In their experience infusion of this fluid was begun at a slow rate (30 ml per hour, 14 g glucose per hour) and within the limits of glucose and fluid tolerance was increased by 10 ml per hour to a maximum of approximately 75–80 ml per hour (3.7 g nitrogen/24 hours, 3500 kcal/24 hours). Insulin requirements were satisfied by adding insulin to the fluid (initially 15 units per bottle, increasing to as much as 50–100 units per bottle).

Despite the apparently favourable results with essential amino acid mixtures in acute renal failure, no differences were seen in

Table 10.8 Parenteral nutrition using essential amino acids only as the nitrogen source. (After [6])

Ingredient	Amount
Water	750 ml
L-amino acids	
Isoleucine	1.4 g
Leucine	2.2 g
Lysine hydrochloride	2.0 g
Methionine	2.2 g
Phenylalanine	2.2 g
Threonine	1.0 g
Tryptophan	0.5 g
Valine	1.6 g
Total	13.1 g
Glucose	350 g
Vitamins	
A	5000 USP units
B1 (thiamine hydrochloride)	25 mg
B2 (riboflavin)	5 mg
B6 (pyridoxine hydrochloride)	7.5 mg
Niacinamide	50 mg
Panthenol	12.5 mg
C (ascorbic acid)	1.5 g
D2 (ergocalciferol)	500 USP units
E (dl-alpha-tocopheryl acetate)	2.5 IU
Calories (non-nitrogen)	1400 Kcal
Osmolarity	2100 mosmol/litre
pH	6.4
Alpha-amino nitrogen	1.3 g
Total nitrogen	1.45 g

blood urea or nitrogen balance when rats with severe experimental uraemia were randomised to receive parenteral nutrition using essential amino acids alone or a complete mixture of essential and non essential amino acids [9]. Moreover, there is no evidence as far as the author is concerned that survival in patients with acute renal failure is significantly higher in those receiving an essential amino acid nitrogen source alone, when compared to those receiving non-essential as well as essential amino acids. For these reasons, we would currently advocate the use of standard L-amino acid nitrogen sources in acute renal failure.

*Metabolic complications of nutritional support
in acute renal failure*

Nutritional support is not to be taken lightly in patients with acute renal failure and very careful monitoring is required. Hyperglycaemia is an inevitable problem and almost all patients require insulin therapy. It is thus important to monitor the serum glucose level frequently, particularly in the beginning. This can be done conveniently at ward level by means of an Ames meter. In our standard parenteral nutrition regimes, we often find it necessary to provide insulin supplements in the form of soluble insulin (1 unit/10 g dextrose) added either to the dextrose containers or the 3 litre delivery bag (see Chapter 8). As stressed by Lee [2, 3], patients with acute renal failure have higher insulin requirements, and he recommends that if 50 ml boluses of 50% dextrose are infused per hour, the insulin requirements will be up to 3 times higher (3 units/10 g dextrose; 75 units/500 ml 50% dextrose).

Apart from the usual electrolyte problems in these patients, hypophosphataemia is a particularly important complication. It often occurs in renal failure patients during parenteral nutrition and should be avoided because many of them are already anaemic, and peripheral tissue oxygenation may be further compromised by hypophosphataemia.

Patient monitoring (Table 10.9)

A full clinical, biochemical, haematological and immunological assessment of nutritional status should be performed before nutritional support is instituted in patients with acute renal failure and base line values should be obtained for all other haematological and biochemical measurements. In practice all such information is usually available since nutritional support has usually been instituted before, acute renal failure developing as a complication of pre-existing problems. The recommendations shown in Table 10.9 should act only as guidelines. The importance of frequent monitoring of glucose electrolyte and phosphate levels has already been stressed.

Nutritional support in patients with established chronic renal failure

Patients with established chronic renal failure are not immune to being subjected to multiple trauma, surgical injury or severe sepsis.

Prior to injury, such patients will have been maintained on either protein restriction (20–40 g protein intake/70 kg 70%

Table 10.9 Monitoring of patients with acute renal failure.

Parameters	Before treatment	Twice daily	Daily	Twice weekly	Weekly
Weight	√				√
Mid-triceps skinfold thickness	√				√
Arm muscle circumference	√				√
Serum albumin	√				√
Serum transferrin	√				√
Lymphocyte count	√				√
Skin tests for candida PPD (tuberculin) Streptokinase Streptodornase	√				√
FBP ESR	√			√	
Serum iron	√				√
Vitamin B12	√				√
Prothrombin time	√		√		
Urinary glucose	√	√			
Blood glucose	√	√			
Electrolytes and urea	√		√		
Creatinine	√		√		
Calcium	√			√	
Phosphate	√			√	
Magnesium	√			√	√
Zinc	√				√
Liver function tests	√				
Blood gases*	√		√		
Extra urinary losses volume electrolytes nitrogen	√		√		
24 hour urinary urea excretion	√		√		

* More or less frequently if indicated

high biological protein, absolute amount dependent on glomerular filtration rates) with or without essential amino acid supplementation (1–2 Rose units) or will have been receiving regular haemodialysis and have a protein intake usually in the region of 1 g protein/kg/day. With proper supervision most of these patients should come close to nitrogen equilibrium, although this may often not be the case, especially if patients fail to ingest their recommended protein intake.

As soon as these patients are subjected to trauma, surgical injury or develop severe sepsis, the whole picture changes. The obligatory catabolism of body protein in response to injury not only places them in negative nitrogen balance, with all the deleterious sequelae, but due to the concomitant release of toxic intracellular substances into the intracellular space, uraemia worsens.

In these circumstances, the principles involved in the nutritional management of their chronic renal failure should be abandoned and instead the principles involved in providing nutritional support in acute renal failure adhered to.

Dialysis requirements

In practical terms, the dialysis requirements of patients with established and controlled chronic renal failure will change in response to injury. Many, who previously have been managed on dietary restriction alone, will require intermittent dialysis and the dialysis requirements of those on regular haemodialysis will increase.

As with patients developing acute renal failure, it is often better to transfer injured patients with chronic renal failure to specialist centres if dialysis facilities do not exist in the referring hospital. In the author's experience, referring physicians persevere with peritoneal haemodialysis for too long in these patients. In relatively inexperienced hands peritoneal dialysis is associated with an unacceptably high incidence of metabolic and infective complications, and as mentioned above, loss of endogenous nitrogen is exacerbated (Table 10.2).

REFERENCES

1 Editorial (1973) Prognosis of acute renal failure. *Br. Med. J.* 1, 435.
2 Lee H.A. (1978) The nutritional management of renal diseases. In *Nutrition in the Clinical Management of Disease*, eds. J.W. Dickerson and H.A. Lee, p. 210. Edward Arnold, London.
3 Lee H.W. (1981) What are the nutritional problems in renal failure? *Acta Chir. Scand.* Suppl 507, 318.

4 Montgomerie J.Z., Kalmanson G.M. & Guze L.B. (1968) Renal failure and infection. *Medicine (Baltimore)* **47**, 1.

5 Abel R.M., Beck C.H., Abbott W.M., Ryan J.A., Barnett G.C. & Fischer J.E. (1973) Improved survival from acute renal failure after treatment with essential L-amino acids and glucose. Results of a prospective double-blind study. *New Engl. J. Med.* **288**, 695.

6 Abel R.M. (1976) Parenteral nutrition in the treatment of renal failure. In *Total Parenteral Nutrition*, ed. J.E. Fischer, p. 1430. Little Brown, Boston.

7 Giordano C. (1963) Use of exogenous and endogenous urea for protein synthesis in normal and uraemic subjects. *J. Lab. Clin. Med.* **62**, 231.

8 Gallina D.L. & Dominquez J.M. (1971) Human utilisation of urea nitrogen in low calorie diets. *J. Nutr.* **101**, 1029.

9 Wennburg A., Denneberg T., Kihlberg R., Kronevi T. & Sterner G. (1981) Effects of total parenteral nutrition in rats with severe experimental uraemia. In *Proceedings 3rd European Congress on Parenteral and Enteral Nutrition*, p 45.

Index

Absorption, physiology of   69–79
Acidosis in starvation   44
Addamal   124, 125, 130, 134
Air embolism   108
Alanine   44
Albumin
  plasma levels
    in monitoring treatment   20
    and nutritional status   15
    and post-operative morbidity   22
  synthesis, in starvation   44
Aminaid   170
Amino acids
  in enteral diet, in liver disease   159–62
  infusions   141
    in acute renal failure   173–5
    in hepatic encephalopathy   153
    post-operative   47, 142
  metabolism, in liver disease   153
Aminofusion L Forte   114
Aminoplex   113, 114
Ammonia, blood levels   152
Anorexia   68
Anthropometric measurements   12
Anticoagulants   108
Arrhythmias   108
Ascorbic acid   63, 64
Aspiration of enteric feeds   96
Assessment, nutritional   9–18
  in parenteral nutrition   140

Bile acids   71
Body mass index   12
Body-weight see Weight
Bone disease in parenteral nutrition   137
Bowel
  disease, inflammatory   34, 81
  pre-operative preparation   81
  see also Short bowel syndrome
Build up   84

Burns
  Energy requirements after   46, 56
  nutritional support in   36, 46, 47

Calcium, nutritional requirements   55, 61
Caloreen   75, 84, 119
Cancer
  gastrointestinal, diets in   81
  nutrition and   31–4
Carbohydrates
  absorption   73
    and enteral nutrition   75
  average daily intake   73
  as energy source   58
    enteral nutrition   75
    parenteral nutrition   115–20, 122
Catecholamines, increase
  in injury   45, 46
  in starvation   44
Catheters   102–13
  checking position   105
  complications   103, 106
  entry site   102, 104
  material for   102, 106
  placement   103, 104
  and sepsis   103, 109–13
Chemotherapy, nutritional support in   33
Chloride
  absorption   78, 79
  nutritional requirements   55
Cholesterol absorption   70
Chromium
  deficiency   62
  nutritional requirement   61
Chylomicrons   72
Clinical pathologists   7
Clinifeed 400   84
Clinifeed Favour   84
Clinifeed-Iso   83, 84
Cobalt, nutritional requirements   61
Coeliac disease, diet in   81

Colitis   35
    ulcerative   35
Copper
    deficiency   61, 62
    nutritional requirements   61
Cortisol production in injury   46
Creatinine, urinary output   13
Creatinine–height index (CHI)   14
Crohn's disease
    diets in   81
    home parenteral nutrition in   141
    magnesium deficiency in   61
    nutritional support in   35, 36
Cyanocobalamine   61, 63

Dialysis, renal   167, 168, 169, 171–3,
    177
Diarrhoea in enteral nutrition   75, 79, 80,
    93, 95
Dieticians   7
Diets
    elemental (predigested)   77, 81, 84, 85
    enteral nutrition   79–85

Electrolyte A   125, 130
Electrolyte B   125, 130
Electrolytes
    abnormalities in enteral nutrition   97
    absorption   78
        and enteral nutrition   79
    nutritional requirements   55, 59
    in parenteral nutrition   124
    see also specific electrolytes
Elemental (predigested) diets   77, 81, 84,
    85
Embolism
    air   108
    pulmonary   108
Encephalopathy
    hepatic   150, 152–63
    Wernicke's   45, 137
Endocarditis, bacterial   108
Endoscopy in tube placement   88
Energy
    expenditure, factors affecting   56
    production
        in injury   46
        in starvation   44
    requirements   55–8
        basic   1, 55
        calculation of   59

Energy requirements (*cont.*)
        hospitalised patients   2
        in injury   46, 56
        in nutritional support   55
        parenteral nutrition   124
        in starvation   44
        after surgery   46, 56
    source
        carbohydrate as   58, 75, 115–20,
            122
        fat as   58, 120–3
            contraindications to   72
        glucose as   59, 115, 122, 123
        in parenteral nutrition   115–23
Ensure   84
Enteral nutrition   51, 68–101
    in acute renal failure   170
    administration
        routes of   68, 85–91
        techniques   91
    benefits   94
    complications   94–8
    diets for   79–85
        contamination of   83, 91, 95, 96
        hospital preparation   82
        prescription of   93
        proprietary   83
    in hepatic encephalopathy   159–62
    nutritional requirements   55
    patient monitoring   98, 160
    starter regimes   93
Essential fatty acids deficiency   123
    in parenteral nutrition   123
    prevention   82
Ethanol as energy source   116, 119

Fat
    absorption   69, 70–2
        and enteral nutrition   72
    emulsions   120, 132
    as energy source   58
        contraindications   72
        in parenteral nutrition   120–3
Fatty acids, essential   *see* Essential fatty
    acids
Feeding
    bags   91, 92
    methods, enteral   68, 85–91
    oral   68, 69, 85
    pumps   91
    tube   69, 87

Fistulae
  enterocutaneous, nutritional support
    in 35
  gastrointestinal, diets in 81
Flexical 84, 85
Fluids
  balance in parenteral nutrition 135
  nutritional requirements 59
  see also Water
Folic acid (folate) 63, 64
  deficiency 136, 137
Fractures and energy expenditure 56
FreAmine II 114
Fructokinase 116, 118
Fructose
  average daily intake 73
  as energy source 116, 117
  metabolism 117

Glucagon increase
  in injury 46
  in starvation 44
Glucokinase 116
Gluconeogenesis 44, 47
Glucoplex 125
Glucose
  energy production from 43, 44
  as energy source 59
    in parenteral nutrition 115, 122,
    123
  intolerance 136
  oligosaccharides 119
Glycerolesterhydrolase 70
Glycogen
  average daily intake 73
  energy production from 43, 44, 45
Glycosuria 136
Grip strength measurement 23
Growth hormone production, in injury 46

Haematinics, deficiency 45
Healing *see* Wound healing
Heparin 108, 111, 130
Hepatic encephalopathy 150, 152–63
Hepatic failure, fulminant 162–3
Hepaticaid 159–62
Hypercalcaemia 64, 138
Hypercalcuria 64, 138
Hyperglycaemia 97, 130, 175
Hyperphosphaturia 138
Hypersensitivity skin testing 16, 20, 22

Hyperuricaemia in starvation 44
Hypokalaemia 60
  in enteral nutrition 97
  in parenteral nutrition 136, 137
Hypophosphataemia 60
  in acute renal failure 175
  in enteral nutrition 97
  in parenteral nutrition 136
Hypoproteinaemia, effects of 2

Immunological system in protein calorie
    malnutrition 16
Infection
  malnutrition and 2, 151
  wound 29, 151
Inflammatory bowel disease 34, 81
Infusion pumps 128
Injury
  metabolic response to 45–7, 48
  nutritional support in 47
Insulin in parenteral nutrition 130, 134,
    136, 175
Intralipid 120, 121, 123, 126–34
Intravenous feeding *see* Parenteral
    nutrition
Iodine, nutritional requirements 61
Iron, nutritional requirements 61
Isocal 83, 84

Jaundice
  cholestatic 138
    diets in 72
  obstructive, diets in 81, 84

Ketone bodies as energy source 44, 45
Kidney disease
  malnutrition in 166
  nutritional management 166–77

Lactase deficiency, enteral diets and 75
Lactose
  absorption 73
  average daily intake 73
  in enteral diets 75
Leukaemias, acute, parenteral nutrition
    in 33
Lipase 70
Liquidised food 68, 69, 85
Liver
  disease
    malnutrition in 150

Liver disease (*cont.*)
    nutritional support in   151–63
  function
    in enteral nutrition   97
    in parenteral nutrition   138
Lymphocyte counts   16, 20, 21

Magnesium
  deficiency   61
    in parenteral nutrition   137
  nutritional requirements   55, 61
Malabsorption   81
  diets in   81
Malnutrition
  definitions   2
  diagnosis   9–20
  in hospitalised patients   1–3
    contributory factors   42
  protein calorie (protein energy, PEM) *see*
    Protein calorie malnutrition
Maltose as energy source   116, 119
Manganese   63
  nutritional requirements   61
Maxijul   84
Metabolic rate
  in injury   45, 46
  in starvation   43
Metabolism, resting, measurement of   55
3-Methylhistidine excretion   15
Micelles, bile salts   71
Midarm muscle circumference (MMC)   13,
    14, 22
Molybdenum   63
  nutritional requirements   61
Multibionta   126, 127, 130, 134
Muscle mass, assessment   13, 14

Nasoduodenal feeding   69, 90
Nasoenteric feeding   90
Nasogastric feeding   69, 87
  disadvantages   37
Nasojejunal feeding   69
Neurological disorders, nutritional support
    in   27
Neurosurgery, nutritional support in   27
Nitrogen
  balance
    energy intake and   56
    monitoring   20
  loss
    in dialysis   168

  in injury   47
    measurement of   48
    support in   48
  measurement of   92
    in injury   48
    in renal failure   167
  nutritional requirements   57
    calculation of   59
    in parenteral nutrition   124
  source
    in enteral nutrition   77, 82, 159–62
    in parenteral nutrition   113, 153–8,
      173–5
Nitrogen sparing effect   121, 122
Nurses, nutrition   7, 111
Nutranel   84, 85
Nutrauxil   84
Nutrient intake, assessment   10
Nutritional support
  expectations for   53
  indications for   27–41
  objectives   52
    limiting factors   54
  post-operative   30
  pre-operative   21, 28–30
  requirements   53–64
  routes   51
    see also Enteral nutrition; Parenteral
      nutrition team   5–8
  aims   5
  composition   6
  role within hospital   7
  see also specific disease states

Oligosaccharides, glucose   119
Osteomalacia   61, 64, 137
Overhydration   135

Pancreatic insufficiency, diet in   72, 77,
    81
Pancreatitis, acute, nutritional support
    in   36
Parenteral nutrition   51, 102–49
  calorie to nitrogen ratios in   124
  delivery systems   126–9, 132
  electrolytes   124
  ending of   140
  energy source   115–23
  home   140
  indications for   52
  metabolic complications   135–8

Parenteral nutrition (*cont.*)
  monitoring 13, 20, 138, 157
  nitrogen source 113
  nutritional requirements 55
  regimes for 128–34
    in acute renal failure 171
    in liver disease 156–9
    prescription for 130, 134
    trace elements 124
    vitamin sources 126
Parentrovite 126, 127, 130, 134
Personnel in nutrition team 6
Phosphate
  nutritional requirements 55, 60
  in parenteral nutrition 130, 136, 138
Phosphofructokinase 16
Pneumothorax, catheters and 108
Potassium
  absorption 78
  deficiency in parenteral nutrition 136
  nutritional requirements 55, 60
Prealbumin, plasma levels 15
Protein
  absorption 76
  and enteral nutrition 77
  energy production from
    in injury 46, 47
    in starvation 44
  stores
    measurements of 14, 23
    and post-operative morbidity 22
  synthesis rates
    indirect measurements of 15
    in injury 47
Protein calorie (energy) malnutrition (PEM)
  associated disease states 28
  clinical consequences 2
  definition 2
  diagnosis 9–20
    composite indices 17
    tests 10–18
      disadvantages of 19
  in liver disease 151, 162
  physical signs 10
  prevention 20, 27
  treatment
    indications for 27
    monitoring 13, 15–17, 20
Pumps
  enteral feeding 91
  infusion 128

Radiotherapy, nutritional support in 33
Regurgitation of enteric feeds 96
Renal failure
  acute, nutritional management in 166–76
  chronic, nutritional support in 176–7
Retinol-binding protein (RBP), plasma levels 15, 22
Rickets 61, 64, 137

Selenium
  deficiency 61, 62
  nutritional requirements 61
Sepsis
  catheters and 103, 109–13
  and energy expenditure 56
  post-operative, hypersensitivity skin tests and 22
Short bowel syndrome, diet and 77, 81
Skin
  testing, hypersensitivity 16, 20, 22
  tunnelling 103
Skinfold measurements 13
Sodium
  absorption 78, 79
  loss, in starvation 44
  nutritional requirements 55, 60
  retention, in injury 47
Solivito 126, 127, 130, 134
Sorbitol
  as energy source 116, 117
  metabolism 117
Starch 73
Starvation
  metabolic responses to 43–5, 48
  nutritional support in 45
Sucrose 73
Surgery
  metabolic response to 45–7
  nutritional support
    post-operative 30, 46, 47
    pre-operative 21, 28–30
  post-operative complications, prediction of 21, 22
Survimed 85
Synthamin 114, 115, 128, 130, 132, 134

Tamponade, cardiac 108
Thiamine 63, 64, 137
Thrombophlebitis 103, 108

Thrombosis, central venous, catheters
    and   106
Thyroxin-binding prealbumin (TBPA),
    plasma levels   15, 22
Trace elements   61–3
  deficiency   62
    in starvation   45
  nutritional requirements   61, 63
  in parenteral nutrition   124, 130, 134
Transferrin, plasma levels
  in monitoring treatment   20
  and nutritional status   15
  and post-operative morbidity   22
Triglycerides
  absorption   70, 72
  energy production from
    in injury   46, 47
    in starvation   44
  use in enteric diets   72
Trisorbon   84
Tube feeding   68, 69. 87
Tubes, feeding
  placement   88
  problems from   94
  types   87
Tumours, effect of nutritional support on
  growth   31
Tunnelling, skin   103

Underhydration   135
Uraemia   172, 173

Vamin N   114
Vanadium   61
Vitamin A   63, 64
  absorption   72
Vitamin B1
  deficiency   64, 137
  requirements   63
Vitamin B12   61, 63
Vitamin C   63, 64
Vitamin D   63, 64
  in parenteral nutrition   137, 138
Vitamins
  deficiencies   64

in parenteral nutrition   137
in protein calorie malnutrition   17
in starvation   45
fat-soluble, absorption of   70, 72
nutritional requirements   63
in parenteral nutrition   126, 130, 134
status, assessment   18
Vitlipid   126, 127, 130, 134
Vivonex   53, 82, 84, 85

Water
  absorption   78
  balance, in parenteral nutrition   135
  loss, in starvation   44
  nutritional requirements   59
  retention, in injury   47
Weight
  gain, in parenteral nutrition   21
  loss
    following injury   47
    following surgery   46, 47
    and post-operative
      morbidity/mortality   21
    in starvation   44
  in nutritional assessment   12
Wernicke–Korsakoff syndrome   64
Wernicke's encephalopathy   45, 137
Wounds
  healing
    malnutrition and   2
    vitamin C and   64
  infection
    liver disease and   151
    pre-operative nutrition and   29

Xylitol
  as energy source   116, 118
  metabolism   118

Zinc
  deficiency   61, 62
    in enteral nutrition   97
    in parenteral nutrition   137
  nutritional requirements   61